SO-EJW-254

David A. Paré, PhD
Glenn Larner
Editors

Collaborative Practice in Psychology and Therapy

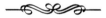
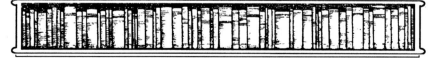

More pre-publication
REVIEWS, COMMENTARIES, EVALUATIONS . . .

"This book weaves critical strands of the best recent innovative work in psychotherapy into a richly textured reflection on how we do our work and an intervention into everyday practice. It provides crucial reference points for practical engagement with the problems that people bring to therapy. The many axes of oppression are addressed by the contributors, in ways that do justice to how these issues are felt and lived, and how they are stored into being. The attention to the social construction of therapeutic practice opens the way for a deconstruction of how we think about the nature of problems. The contributors bring therapeutic and research skills from many disciplines and an urgent sense that all good therapy needs to be theoretically enriched and linked to the best traditions of action research. The book opens the way for reconceptualizing how therapy can become a space not only for interpreting the world but also for changing it."

Ian Parker, PhD
Editor, *Deconstructing Psychotherapy;*
Professor of Psychology,
Manchester Metropolitan University,
United Kingdom

"With *Collaborative Practice in Psychology and Therapy,* David Paré and Glenn Larner, along with authors from around the world, have crafted a far-ranging text. Organized around the metaphor of 'knowing-with,' rather than 'knowing that,' the book explores postmodern psychology in the realms of theory, practice, supervision, and research. Beginning with a number of chapters from oft-quoted theoreticians, the book then moves to practice ideas. The authors invite us into consulting rooms, schools, and organizations, sharing ideas about collaborative relationships that are at once practical and groundbreaking. The chapters on research are inspiring and thought-provoking, and the chapters on supervision have brought a new sense of possibility to my own work as a supervisor."

Jill Freedman, MSW
Co-Director,
Evanston Family Therapy Center,
Evanston, IL

The Haworth Clinical Practice Press
An Imprint of The Haworth Press, Inc.
New York • London • Oxford

Collaborative Practice
in Psychology and Therapy

HAWORTH Practical Practice in Mental Health
Lorna L. Hecker, PhD
Senior Editor

101 Interventions in Family Therapy edited by Thorana S. Nelson and Terry S. Trepper

101 More Interventions in Family Therapy edited by Thorana S. Nelson and Terry S. Trepper

The Practical Practice of Marriage and Family Therapy: Things My Training Supervisor Never Told Me by Mark Odell and Charles E. Campbell

The Therapist's Notebook for Families: Solution-Oriented Exercises for Working with Parents, Children, and Adolescents by Bob Bertolino and Gary Schultheis

The Therapist's Notebook for Children and Adolescents: Homework, Handouts, and Activities for Use in Psychotherapy edited by Catherine Ford Sori and Lorna L. Hecker

The Therapist's Notebook for Lesbian, Gay, and Bisexual Clients: Homework, Handouts, and Activities for Use in Psychotherapy edited by Joy S. Whitman and Cynthia J. Boyd

Collaborative Practice in Psychology and Therapy edited by David A. Paré and Glenn Larner

A Guide to Self-Help Workbooks for Mental Health Clinicians and Researchers by Luciano L' Abate

Resources in Prevention, Psychotherapy, and Rehabilitation for Clinicians and Researchers edited by Luciano L'Abate

Collaborative Practice in Psychology and Therapy

David A. Paré, PhD
Glenn Larner
Editors

The Haworth Clinical Practice Press
An Imprint of The Haworth Press, Inc.
New York • London • Oxford

Published by

The Haworth Clinical Practice Press, an imprint of The Haworth Press, Inc., 10 Alice Street, Binghamton, NY 13904-1580.

Cover design by Lora Wiggins.

Library of Congress Cataloging-in-Publication Data

Collaborative practice in psychology and therapy / David A. Paré, Glenn Larner, editors.
    p. cm.
  Includes bibliographical references and index.
  ISBN 0-7890-1785-7 (hard : alk. paper)—ISBN 0-7890-1786-5 (soft : alk. paper)
  1. Social psychiatry. 2. Social psychology. I. Paré, David A. II. Larner, Glenn.
RC455.C612 2003
362.2—dc21
                                 2003001593

To Pete 'n Anne
From David

To Liz, Mat, and Tim
From Glenn

CONTENTS

RESEARCH: EXPLORING FROM WITHIN— COLLABORATIVE RESEARCH PRACTICES

ABOUT THE EDITORS

David Paré, PhD, is an assistant professor and counselor educator in the Faculty of Education at the University of Ottawa, Canada. He is co-director of The Glebe Institute, A Centre for Constructive and Collaborative Practice, which offers therapy services, training, and supervision in Ottawa. Dr. Paré has published and presented widely on the subject of collaborative and discursive therapies. His writings have appeared in *Family Process,* the *Journal of Collaborative Therapy,* and the *Canadian Journal of Counselling.* He has also contributed to *The Therapist's Notebook* (Haworth) and *The Therapist's Notebook for Children and Adolescents* (Haworth).

Glenn Larner is a senior clinical psychologist and family therapist in Australia with more than twenty-five years of experience in child and adolescent therapy. He has published widely on the topic of deconstruction and therapy, including a contribution to *Deconstructing Psychotherapy,* and is an associate editor for the *Australian and New Zealand Journal of Family Therapy.*

Contributors

Jon K. Amundson, PhD, is a chartered psychologist who has been in independent practice in Calgary, Alberta, Canada, since 1980. Aside from developing a clinical approach characterized by brief time frames and defined outcomes, Jon has written and published on topics ranging from ethical behavior and professional conduct to family therapy, psychological diagnosis, and divorce mediation. His writings have appeared in *Family Process,* the *Journal of Systemic Therapies,* the *Dulwich Centre Newsletter,* and many other publications.

The Anti-Harassment Team at Selwyn College in Auckland, New Zealand, is a collection of young women and men committed to creatively countering the negative impact of harassment and other destructive school behaviors. The team has contributed to a number of publications as well as presented its work in New Zealand and Australia.

Aileen Cheshire, BA, Diploma Teaching, Diploma Guidance, Master of Counseling, has an extensive work history in school counseling. Her current work combines private practice with counselor education. She has published a number of articles in the *Dulwich Centre Newsletter* and contributed a chapter to *Narrative Therapy in Practice: The Archaeology of Hope* (Jossey-Bass, 1996). In 2000, she received a Winston Churchill Fellowship Award with Dorothea Lewis for their outstanding work with the Anti-Harassment Team at Selwyn College in Auckland, New Zealand.

Kathie Crocket, PhD, teaches counseling in the Department of Human Development and Counseling at the University of Waikato, Hamilton, New Zealand. She is a co-editor of *Narrative Therapy in Practice: The Archaeology of Hope* (Jossey-Bass, 1996). Kathie's doctoral research investigated the implications of the narrative metaphor for counseling supervision.

Robert Doan, PhD, is a full professor at the University of Central Oklahoma in Edmond, Oklahoma, where he teaches master's-level classes in counseling and marriage and family therapy. His articles have appeared in a number of journals, and he is co-author, along with Alan Parry, of *Story Re-Visions: Narrative Therapy in a Postmodern World.*

John Drury, PhD, has current research interests including empowerment in collective action, constructions of and reactions to "deviance," and the discursive construction of "otherness" and pathology in intergroup relations. His doctoral research on crowd dynamics and identity change was carried out under the supervision of Steve Reicher at the University of Exeter, United Kingdom. After earning his doctorate, he worked for a year as a researcher with the Trust for the Study of Adolescence, Brighton, United Kingdom, looking at youth communication. He currently is lecturer in social psychology at the University of Sussex, United Kingdom, where he also teaches courses on group processes, discourse analysis, and the relation between social psychology and social policy.

Kevin Fitzsimmons, MSW, and **Larry Zucker, MSW,** developed and direct the Resource-Oriented Therapy Training Program, a year-long immersion in postmodern therapies at the Southern California Counseling Center. Both are on the family therapy faculty at the Counseling Center, instructors in the Master's of Psychology program at Antioch University, Los Angeles, and in private practice. In addition, they have provided many workshops in narrative and solution-oriented approaches to therapy. Kevin also teaches part time at the UCLA Graduate School of Social Work. Kevin's most recent publication is a chapter on the bias of the helping professions against multicultural clients in *Controversial Issues in Multiculturalism* (Allyn & Bacon, 1996) edited by Diane De Anda. Larry is currently working with Clean Slate, a low-fee program offering tattoo removal and counseling to support gang members in changing their relationships with their communities.

Stephen Frosh, PhD, is a professor of psychology and the director of the Centre for Psychosocial Studies in the School of Psychology at Birkbeck College, University of London. He formerly was a consultant clinical psychologist and vice dean in the Child and Family Department of the Tavistock Clinic, London, England. His numerous academic publications include *For and Against Psychoanalysis* (Routledge, 1997), *Sexual Difference: Masculinity and Psychoanalysis* (Routledge, 1994), *Identity Crisis: Modernity, Psychoanalysis and the Self* (Macmillan, 1991), *The Politics of Psychoanalysis* (Macmillan, 1987; Second Edition, 1999), and *Child Sexual Abuse* (with Danya Glaser, Second Edition, Macmillan, 1993). He is co-editor with Anthony Elliott of *Psychoanalysis in Contexts* (Routledge, 1995). His most recent book is *Young Masculinities: Understanding Boys in Contemporary Society,* with Ann Phoenix and Rob Pattman (Palgrave, 2002).

Heather Gridley, MA, is a senior lecturer in the Department of Psychology at Victoria University, Melbourne, Australia, where she coordinates one of only two Australian postgraduate programs in community psychology. Heather is an active researcher in Melbourne's West, a culturally diverse, industrialized region whose residents have typically lacked access to resources and services supportive of healthy communities. She trained as a counseling/clinical psychologist, but her interest in community psychology stemmed from her work in community health, in which she became aware of the limitations of interventions directed solely at individuals. Heather's teaching, research, and practice are based on feminist principles, and in 1995 she received the Australian Psychological Society's Elaine Dignan Award for significant contributions concerning women and psychology. A Fellow of the Australian Psychological Society, she has held national positions in both the College of Community Psychologists and Women and Psychology Interest Group and has served two terms on the APS Board of Directors.

David J. Harper, PhD, is a senior lecturer in clinical psychology on the Professional Doctorate in Clinical Psychology program at the University of East London, United Kingdom. He was a co-author of *Deconstructing Psychopathology* (Sage, 1995) and has published a number of papers exploring the use of qualitative, deconstructive, and broadly social constructionist approaches to the concepts of "paranoia" and "delusion."

Arlene Katz, EdD, is an instructor in the Department of Social Medicine at Harvard Medical School. As director of the Community

Councils Project at the Cambridge Health Alliance, she worked with colleagues and community elders to develop a Council of Elders to teach health care trainees about the lived experience of aging, which has been effective in addressing ageism and emphasizing relationally responsive care. This is one of a series of dialogically structured projects involving the development of "resourceful communities" to increase health care professionals' sense of accountability to those they serve. Dr. Katz has authored many articles on mentoring, poetic practices, and collaborative methods of care, research, and training and has consulted and lectured on these subjects nationally and internationally.

Dorothea Lewis, MA, MCouns, is a school counselor and counselor educator in Auckland, New Zealand. Her work with Aileen Cheshire and the Anti-Harassment Team at Selwyn College has received international attention. Dorothea has published a number of articles about her collaborative practices. She received a Winston Churchill Fellowship Award in 2000 for her work with the Anti-Harassment Team.

Jill C. Manning, MSc, RSW, is a marital and family therapist who currently resides and practices in Edmonton, Alberta, Canada. She completed a bachelor of arts in communications studies at the University of Calgary, a master of science in marital and family therapy from Loma Linda University, and in 1994 studied international relations at the Jerusalem Center for Near Eastern Studies in Israel. Jill completed a clinical internship in the Family Therapy Program at the University of Calgary, and it was here that she met and was supervised by Dr. Alan Parry. Experiences as a missionary in France and California greatly influenced her career path and interest in postmodernism.

Wally McKenzie, MSocSci, is a private counseling practitioner who presents internationally on the subject of narrative therapy. He has co-authored two book chapters, and his work also appears on public Web sites devoted to collaborative therapy practices such as <www.planet-therapy.com> and <www.narrativeapproaches.com>. In addition, Wally teaches counseling in the master's in counseling programs at both the University of Waikato and Unitech in New Zealand. He is codirector of the Hamilton Therapy Centre, Hamilton, New Zealand.

Donald McMenamin, PhD, is a school counselor in Hamilton, New Zealand. His innovative and collaborative counseling practices have been detailed in the *Dulwich Centre Newsletter.* Donald is a consultant in two projects funded by the New Zealand Ministry of Education that aim to implement restorative justice practices to reduce school suspensions for both mainstream populations and for Maori (indigenous) students.

Sheila McNamee, PhD, is a professor of communication at the University of New Hampshire and holds the university's Class of 1944 Professorship. She also is a founding member of the Taos Institute <www.taosinstitute.org>. Her work is focused on transformation within a variety of social and institutional contexts including organizations, education, health care, psychotherapy, and communities. She is author of *Relational Responsibility: Resources for Sustainable Dialogue,* with Kenneth Gergen (Sage, 1998). Her other books include *Therapy As Social Construction,* with Kenneth Gergen (Sage, 1992), *Philosophy in Therapy: The Social Poetics of Therapeutic Conversation,* with Klaus Deissler (Carl Auer Systeme Verlag, 2000), and *The Appreciative Organization,* with the Taos Institute Founders (2001). Professor McNamee has also authored numerous articles and chapters on social constructionist theory and practice, which she actively uses in a variety of contexts to bring communities of participants with diametrically opposing viewpoints together to create liveable futures. Professor McNamee lectures and consults regularly, both nationally and internationally, for universities, private institutes, organizations, and communities.

Geoffrey Nelson, PhD, is a professor of psychology and former director of the master's program in community psychology at Wilfrid Laurier University. Professor Nelson has obtained numerous research grants and contracts and has published widely in two research areas: issues related to psychiatric consumer/survivors (housing, social support, community mental health programs, family stress, self-help/mutual aid) and primary prevention programs for children in the school and neighborhood context. For six years, he served as the senior editor of the *Canadian Journal of Community Mental Health,* and in 1999 he received the Harry V. McNeill Award for Innovation in Community Mental Health from the Society for Community Research and Action and the American Psychological Foundation.

Alan Parry, PhD, is a psychologist who practices family therapy at the Family Therapy Program at the University of Calgary. He obtained his PhD in religion and social psychology in the late 1960s at Berkeley and has never quite recovered. He could not stop telling stories about life in the 1960s and so became a narrative therapist as a way of externalizing this habit. He also wrote articles about narrative therapy and chaos theory in a further attempt to control himself, even co-authoring *Story Re-Visions: Narrative Therapy in the Postmodern World* with his friend Robert Doan, another refugee from that era. He is currently working on a project titled *Wittgenstein's Therapy: The Performative Way.*

Isaac Prilleltensky, PhD, is a professor of human and organizational development at Peabody College of Vanderbilt University. Prior to that he was a professor of psychology at Victoria University in Melbourne, Australia, where he also was the director of the Wellness Promotion Unit. He is the author of *The Morals and Politics of Psychology: Psychological Discourse and the Status Quo* (State University of New York Press, 1994); co-author with Geoff Nelson of *Doing Psychology Critically: Making a Difference in Diverse Settings* (Palgrave, 2002); and co-editor of both *Critical Psychology* (Sage, 1997) and *Promoting Family Wellness and Preventing Child Maltreatment* (University of Toronto Press, 2001). Isaac is currently collaborating with Geoffrey Nelson on a new community psychology textbook to be published by Palgrave. Isaac is a fellow of the Division of Community Psychology of the American Psychological Association, and in 2002 he was a Visiting Fellow of the British Psychological Society. In 2001 he was the recipient of Victoria University's Vice-Chancellor's Excellence in Research Award. He is interested in the promotion of value-based practice and interventions in community mental health. He believes that social justice is a key value in the prevention of psychological problems and in the promotion of personal, relational, and collective wellness.

Lois Shawver, PhD, is a clinical psychologist in private practice who supervises graduate and postdoctoral students in clinical psychology. In addition to publishing numerous articles on postmodernism and psychoanalysis, Lois is author of *And the Flag Was Still There: Straight People, Gay People, and Sexuality in the U.S. Military.* She serves on the editorial board for the *American Journal of Psychoanalysis* and for the journal *New Therapist.* Lois also leads discussion within a high-profile online community of professionals devoted to the discussion of postmodern issues as they relate to therapy.

John Shotter, PhD, is a professor of interpersonal relations in the Department of Communication, University of New Hampshire. His long-term interest is in the social conditions conducive to people having a voice in the development of participatory democracies and civil societies. John's extensive writings make him one of the premier articulators of social constructionist philosophy. His recent books include *Cultural Politics of Everyday Life: Social Constructionism, Rhetoric, and Knowing of the Third Kind* (University of Toronto, 1993) and *Conversational Realities: The Construction of Life Through Language* (Sage, 1993).

Craig Smith, PhD, is a marriage, family, and child counselor in private practice at the Solana Beach Counseling Center in San Diego County. He also teaches counselors at San Diego State University, supervises at various local agencies, and does trainings in collaborative therapy. Craig is co-editor of *Narrative Therapies with Children and Adolescents* (Guilford, 1997) with Dave Nylund.

Tom Strong, PhD, CPsych, is a counselor-educator and assistant professor in the Division of Applied Psychology at the University of Calgary. Tom's writing focuses on the theory, ethics, and pragmatics of discursive practice in health conversations and psychotherapy. Tom is co-editor (with David Paré) of the forthcoming book *Furthering Talk: Advances in the Discursive Therapies.* He also is a faculty member with the Discursive Therapies Program of Massey University, New Zealand, a contributing editor to *New Therapist,* and a connoisseur of fine roots music.

Carla Willig, PhD, is a lecturer in psychology in the Department of Psychology at City University, London. She is also a member of the editorial boards of the *Journal of Health Psychology* and *Psychology and Health*. Carla has published numerous articles and book chapters and is editor of *Applied Discourse Analysis: Social and Psychological Interventions* (Open University Press, 1999), and one of the authors of *Health Psychology: Theory, Research and Practice* (Sage, 2000). She has also published a book, *Introducing Qualitative Research in Psychology: Adventures in Theory and Methods* (University Press, 2001).

Foreword

The past several decades of postmodern scholarship have brought forth profound reflection on the otherwise comfortable and nurturing traditions of Western culture. No longer do such terms as *truth, objectivity, knowledge, rationality,* and *progress* enjoy a commanding presence. As many find, the very deployment of such terms carries with it a subtle but insidious shroud of suppression, a silencing of voices, an obliteration of diversity, and a closure of dialogue. Also, new and important challenges have been mounted to existing structures of authority: who has the right to declare the real or to proclaim the good for all? If there are no foundations for such claims, what is the purpose of authority and the function of our structures of power beyond self-service? Finally, with these challenges has come a deep questioning of the bounded self— the concept of a rational and self-directing agent—pivotal to our traditional institutions of education and law, and central to our practices of organizational life, mental health, and everyday morality. If such a concept is deeply flawed, then what are we to make of these institutions and practices? Are they not open as well to serious question?

These various domains of critical reflection set the stage for enormous liberation. All the taken-for-granted truths of the past are thrust into contingency; all normal practices of daily life are opened to reassessment; we are freed from the constraints of tradition to consider new and perhaps more promising potentials. However, recognizing the threshold of liberation is one thing; crossing over into new territory is quite another. Recognizing the limits of our traditions is not necessarily to abandon them—we can step out of history no more than we can step over our own shadows. What should be retained, what are the most promising targets of transformation, how are we to proceed, and why?

These have been challenging questions for social science scholars and practitioners in particular, for they have long been harbingers of hope for a better society. For those caught up in the challenges of postmodernism, the initial and now the most well-developed initiative has been critical in posture. The broadscale critique of modernism enabled a new range of critical tools to be honed, and these have now become vital elements in building a critically reflexive science (e.g., Fox and Prilleltensky, 1997; Holdstock, 2000).

Yet although continuing critique is essential, many have also seen this stance as limited. Again, it is one thing to become conscious of flawed assumptions and practices, but if this is our singular posture we remain locked in combat without the development of new visions. Slowly, new visions have emerged, and these have given rise to an exciting array of adventures. In the case of social science inquiry, there is a now a burgeoning literature on discourse (e.g., Edwards and Potter, 1992), the historical construction of the person (Danziger, 1997), the cultural lodgment of psychological process (Bruner, 1990), the communal basis of memory (Middleton and Edwards, 1990), the narrative construction of lives (Josselson and Lieblich, 1993), and much more. These new lines of inquiry are matched as well by a vital flourishing of new methods of research. Denzin and Lincoln's (2001) voluminous *Handbook of Qualitative Research* harbors a treasure of new developments, and Reason and Bradbury's (2001) *Handbook of Action Research* represents a bold step toward reconstructing methodology. These developments are also matched by innovations in conceptual domains. Much of my own work of the past decade (Gergen, 1994, 1999, 2001) has been concerned with developing metatheoretical resources for a revitalized social science, and forging theory that moves beyond the individual as the fundamental atom of concern to relational process.

Work in all these areas has also proceeded in active dialogue with practitioners in numerous domains. For example, the moves toward narrative (McLeod, 1997), brief therapy (de Shazer, 1994), and postmodern therapy (Anderson, 1997) are all illustrative examples of the ways in which postmodern sensitivities have inspired change in therapeutic practice. Further, in the pedagogical sphere, educators have pursued ways of fostering more collaborative, dialogic, and democratic practices in the classroom (Bruffee, 1993; Rogoff, Turkanis, and Bartlett, 2001). Organizational specialists have developed similar forms of practice for transforming organizations (Cooperrider et al., 1999), and community change agents have similarly generated discursively conscious means of ameliorating conflict (Chasin et al., 1996).

It is also interesting to note that, owing primarily to the liberatory influence of much postmodern writing, scholars and practitioners have also begun to challenge disciplinary boundaries. The traditional chasms of communication separating the various disciplines and driving a wedge between theorists and practitioners increasingly seem both arbitrary and stultifying. The result of such questioning has been a burgeoning of creative cross-talk and rich new ventures that animate mind, spirit, and action. We find, for example, initiatives that explore the significance of Foucault for social workers (Chambon, Irving, and Epstein, 1999), the aesthetic and literary dimensions of ethnography (Bochner and Ellis, 2002), the ethical implications of relational discourse (McNamee and Gergen, 1999), and the implications of social constructionism for theology (Hermans et al., 2002) among them.

Yet these are but bare beginnings into the new territory of unimaginable potential, and it is at just this point that the present work gains singular significance. In my view the editors of this book, David Paré and Glenn Larner, take seriously the postmodern replacement of truth with pragmatic impact as the criterion of effective science. They appropriately see that social theory and research is of significance to the culture not because it reveals the truth but because of the way in which life is made intelligible and actions are celebrated or condemned. Further, they understand very well that judgments concerning the pragmatic impact of theory and research are inevitably wedded to values and politics; we cannot proceed without abiding concern with the forms of life that we create with our actions—as researchers, therapists, teachers, and so on. Finally, Paré and Larner see very clearly the limits of the individualist tradition of understanding and practice, and they appreciate the enormously important implications of deliberating and acting relationally.

It is within this context that the present book has emerged. The participants in this text—all of whom share the concerns of the editors—were invited to push the envelope. In effect, participants were invited to describe their present trajectories in terms of theory and inquiry, and discuss the differences these developments make to current practices. Or again, in terms of practice, "describe the innovations in which you have been engaged, share your successes, and tell us of their implications for both theoretical understanding and professional life."

In my view the contributors answered the call by providing imaginative, passionate, and carefully deliberated accounts from the frontier. Several closely related themes particularly struck me as I read through these chapters. The first is a deep distrust of what might be called the tradition of monologic knowing. Whether therapist, counselor, educator, or other, so many of these authors see expert knowledge (truth claims, paradigmatic commitments, or beliefs in rational or moral superiority) as diminishing the possibilities for human flexibility and change. Here the various reactions to this suspicion are illuminating. For in so many of the chapters we not only find ways to circumvent monologic knowing but to honor the client, student, trainee, or others engaged in forms of practice. The second intriguing theme resonates with the first. Many of these contributors find in the practice of collaboration a powerful means of creative change. It is not simply that collaboration opens a space for participation, but rather that the outcome of effective collaboration enables the participants—both practitioners and those they serve—to move into new spaces of understanding and action. Finally, I became acutely aware that these various incursions into collaborative space carried with them strong moral and political investments. The contributors did not apologize for their valuative positions, nor did they attempt to ground them in some foundational logic or ethic. Rather, they let us know that in working *with* as opposed to *on* those we serve, we establish what might be called a "process ethics," or "process politics." The nature of the good society is not in this way specified; this would be a form of monologic knowledge. Rather, as the collaborative process is set in motion, new visions and values may emerge that reflect the engagement of all participants. It is my fond hope that future readers of this work will share the fascination and illumination I found in these pages.

Kenneth J. Gergen

REFERENCES

Anderson, H. (1997). *Conversation, language, and possibilities: A postmodern approach to psychotherapy.* New York: Basic Books.

Bochner, A.P. and Ellis, C. (Eds.) (2002). *Ethnographically speaking.* Walnut Creek, CA: Altamira.

Bruffee, K. (1993). *Collaborative learning*. Baltimore, MD: Johns Hopkins University Press.

Bruner, J. (1990). *Acts of meaning*. Cambridge, MA: Harvard University Press.

Chambon, A.S., Irving, A., and Epstein, L. (Eds.) (1999). *Reading Foucault for social work*. New York: Cambridge University Press.

Chasin, R., Herzig, M., Roth, S., Chasin, L., Becker, C., and Stains, R. (1996). From diatribe to dialogue on divisive public issues: Approaches drawn from family therapy. *Mediation Quarterly* 13:323-344.

Cooperrider, D., Sorensen, P., Whitney, D., and Yaeger, T. (Eds) (1999). *Appreciative inquiry*. Cleveland, OH: Stipes.

Danziger, K. (1997). *Naming the mind*. Thousand Oaks, CA: Sage.

de Shazer, S. (1994). *Words were originally magic*. New York: Norton.

Denzin, N. and Lincoln, Y. (Eds.) (2001). *Handbook of qualitative research*. Thousand Oaks, CA: Sage.

Edwards, D. and Potter, J. (1992). *Discursive psychology*. London: Sage.

Fox, D. and Prilleltensky, I. (Eds.) (1997). *Critical psychology: An introduction*. London: Sage.

Gergen, K.J. (1994). *Realities and relationships*. Cambridge, MA: Harvard University Press.

Gergen, K.J. (1999). *An invitation to social construction*. London: Sage.

Gergen, K.J. (2001). Psychological science in a postmodern context. *American Psychologist* 56(10):803-813.

Hermans, C.A.M., Immink, G., de Jong, A., and van der Lans, J. (Eds.) (2002). *Social constructionism and theology*. Leiden, The Netherlands: Brill.

Holdstock, T.L. (2000). *Re-examining psychology: Critical perspectives and African insights*. London: Routledge.

Josselson, R. and Lieblich, A. (Eds.) (1993). *The narrative study of lives*. Thousand Oaks, CA: Sage.

McLeod, J. (1997). *Narrative and psychotherapy*. London: Sage.

McNamee, S. and Gergen, K.J. (1999). *Relational responsibility*. Thousand Oaks, CA: Sage.

Middleton, D. and Edwards, D. (Eds.) (1990). *Collective remembering*. London: Sage.

Reason, P. and Bradbury, H. (Eds.) (2001). *Handbook of action research*. London: Sage.

Rogoff, B., Turkanis, C.G., and Bartlett, L. (Eds.) (2001). *Learning together: Children and adults in a school community*. New York: Oxford University Press.

Acknowledgments

From David Paré

Books such as this emerge from communities, and I would like to take the opportunity to thank a range of people from those communities—near and far, recently and in the past—who have contributed to this book's appearance in the world.

First, the theorists and practitioners whose work I initially regarded from a distance, who ignited passion that has not abated, and who have now become colleagues with shared commitments. Thanks to Michael White and David Epston for their courageous and visionary contributions to this field, and for the Dulwich Centre community that continues to creatively expand on narrative ideas and practices. Thanks to the core of compassionate educators who shaped the innovative counseling program at the University of Waikato in Hamilton, New Zealand: Gerald Monk, John Winslade, Wendy Drewery, Kathie Crocket, and Wally McKenzie. My time with them—the laughs and the learning—continues to reverberate as I continue on my journey.

Thanks also to Alan Jenkins and Ken Gergen, with whom I have crossed paths less often. Their work has helped me to locate myself within the room and within the field. Alan's clinical clarity is a beacon; Ken's ability to pull together the threads of a vast tapestry is a gift to the community.

Thanks to Don Sawatzky for his steady guidance during my early training, and for opening the door to a world of theory and practice that has added so much richness to my life. And thanks also to the Lousage Institute community in Edmonton that steadfastly supported me in my first uncertain steps.

Some of the energy that produced this book I gained from colleagues whose enthusiasm for alternative practices have invigorated me over the years: Ninetta Tavano, Craig Smith, Mary Anne Rombach, and Tom Strong. Thanks to them all, and thanks to Mishka Lysack, my codirector at the Glebe Institute, for his commitment, focus, and unwavering patience.

This book came to The Haworth Press through Series Editor Lorna Hecker of Purdue University. Thanks go to Lorna for her interest in seeing new and sometimes challenging ideas spoken in plain talk, and for giving Glenn and I the elbow room to work with our many talented contributors.

Thanks, too, to Jasmine Albagli and Eun Jin Kim. Jasmine, you restored order when chaos descended, and always with good humor. Eun Jin, you never blinked in the face of a frequently overcrowded agenda.

In a venture devoted to the quest for relational nonviolence, I could not have asked for a better collaborator than Glenn Larner. From a few fleeting hallway chats between then-strangers at a conference in Sydney, Australia, Glenn and I forged a working relationship separated by oceans. Many hundreds of e-mails and the occasional phone chat later, we have arrived at the completion of this project, cyber-relationship fully intact. My thanks to Glenn, who enacts the values he so eloquently writes about.

Finally, my gratitude goes out to the folks who have endured me and sustained me through this enterprise over the past three years. Thanks to Susan, Casey, and Liam: they make it worth it.

From Glenn Larner

David has said it all for me and I thank him for his patience, dedication, and encouragement in finishing this project. I also join him in dedicating this book to the many mentors and colleagues in narrative and family therapy, such as Max Cornwell, who as editor of the *Australian and New Zealand Journal of Family Therapy* first invited me to publish an article, and Carmel Flaskas, who supervised my work and inspired systemic thinking in therapy.

I would also like to acknowledge John Kaye, who arranged several conferences "down under" in Adelaide on the postmodern social construction of knowledge. There I had the opportunity to hear and meet key figures in the field, such as Ian Parker, who invited me to contribute a chapter to a wider conversation on deconstruction and therapy. Thanks also must go to the critical psychology mob at Western Sydney for arranging an inaugural world conference where I briefly met David and proposed out of the blue that we write something together.

This is deconstruction in action, on the margin or outside the lecture halls. And of course Derrida has been my inspiration in thinking about such notions, such as hospitality and a dialogue between the modern and postmodern, which this book attempts to reflect.

Introduction

Toward an Ethic of Hospitality

David A. Paré
Glenn Larner

The past three decades have seen a series of provocative reflections (e.g., Caputo, 1997; Foucault, 1980; Habermas, 1972; Lyotard, 1984; Rorty, 1979) on the long-standing Western tradition of privileging institutional knowledge and holding it up as the royal standard, the unassailable truth to vanquish all pretenders to the throne. In effect, these and countless other voices have expressed dissent with what Weber (1987) calls "*imposability,* the conditions under which arguments, categories, and values impose and maintain a certain authority" (p. 18). That authority is not inclined to self-examination; it speaks with certainty and acts with resolve. It expresses itself as professional "expertise" which excludes, if not outright rejects, alternate points of view.

In the institution of psychology, the recent reevaluation of the expert-oriented stance has generated an exhilarating range of ideas for approaching practice with an openness to mutual exploration and discovery. There is a make-it-up-together spirit, a shift from *im*posing to *com*posing, accompanied by a rejuvenated vocabulary of *coconstructed meanings* and *dialogic mutuality*. This book seeks to further the quest for self-reflective and collaborative practice while acknowledging the challenges that quest presents.

And there *are* challenges. One of these relates to the temptation to abandon a collaborative ethic when the going gets tough—to slip back into a "fix-it" mode, thereby sacrificing relationship at the altar of technique. It is far easier to speak on behalf of mutuality than to embody it in the complex, changeful, and challenging realm of practice. The clinicians, teachers, supervisors, and researchers who have contributed to this book were asked to share some of the specific approaches they have developed which align their commitment to mutuality in relationships with what they actually *do* from day to day in their work. Staying that course requires clarity of vision and moral commitment. This is true of the microexchanges of therapy, training, supervision, and research where professional hubris, weariness with uncertainty, or plain desperation may lead us to unilaterally legislate structures and frameworks. It is also true of the broader conversation that is theory, and therein lies a second challenge.

The creative explorations associated with postmodern psychology are frequently accompanied by a dismissal of previous accounts of human experience—a dismissal that ironically duplicates the dualistic, us-versus-them ideology it purports to critique. As Kenneth Gergen (1999) points out, critical tools play a vital role in identifying concerns, but the object of a critique of the modern Western tradition in psychology "is not to argue for abandoning these traditions. Rather it is to open the commonplace to critical inspection and to explore the possibility of fresh and more viable alternatives" (p. 19). So a second key aim of this book is to present theory as a generative resource. Although the theoretical contributions discussed here are much influenced by the grand conversation that is postmodernism, they are dedicated more to pointing a way forward than trumping the claims of modernism. In that respect, they are guides for practice.

The traditional separation of theory from practice begins to break down when one assumes, as do the contributors gathered here, that speaking and writing are crafts of world making (Bruner, 1987; Paré, 2001) which effect telling change through the shaping of human understanding and action. This formidable enterprise is inevitably a social process, an act of relationship. The principal aim of this book, then, is to explore ways of speaking the world into being that do not do violence to others. This refers to the potential violence of theory, authority, expertise, and technology to override others' contributions to their life narratives (Larner, 1999). Those "others" include therapeutic clients, students, and supervisees; research participants; and also you, the reader. Beyond the domains of "theoretical constructs" or "clinical interventions," this collection of essays seeks to engage you with ideas and practices in a manner that does not perpetuate relational violence.

To this end, the contributors advocate for a collaborative knowing—a *knowing-with*—which can be contrasted with a long epistemological tradition of describing that which is purported to be real and true, the *knowing-that* (Paré, 1999; Polkinghorne, 1993; Shotter, 1993), which permeates the psychology literature. The knowing-that position is much like the stance of the colonizer, brandishing The Word to the unwashed masses (Todd and Wade, 1994). The paradox here is that to *know* one cannot avoid taking some position; but the key is whether knowledge is held heavily rather than lightly, to use one of Milan Kundera's well-known metaphors. The stance we encourage here places dialogue before didacticism. It involves openness to dialogue as one engages in practice and in the description of practice (which, as noted previously, can be understood as practice itself). Our preferred orientation is therefore one of what Cornell (1992) has called "institutional humility": we invite a consideration of collaborative alternatives without buttressing them with refutations of previous perspectives and practices. By striving to make explicit the *practice* of collaborative knowing, we hope to offer those of a different persuasion a greater degree of freedom in choosing their own positioning. This actualizes the moral thrust of nonoppositional, noncolonizing knowing by encouraging dialogue between therapists and psychologists expressing a diversity of opinions, a process that can only enrich the field.

Collaborative Practice in Psychology and Therapy engages with these timely questions in four central domains of psychology: theory, therapy practice, teaching/supervision, and research. It suggests ways of moving the whole field forward in a manner that creates space for many voices, and is vigilant of the ethical responsibility of wielding knowledge in the service of others. In a nutshell, the book advocates for a view of all psychological practice as relationship characterized by the mutual exchange of knowledge and meaning. The chapters provide readers with a range of examples of clinical, research, training, and supervisory practices in psychology and therapy that mindfully seek to avoid the fundamentalist zeal that characterizes many versions of both modern and postmodern psychology.

We have included a broad spectrum of theorists and professionals from a range of designated "camps." The trumpeting of one brand of psychology and therapy over another tends to promote an antagonistic dynamic which, in its own way, can be understood as theoretically violent. We would like this book to honor reflexivity and multiplicity; many roads lead to Rome. We believe that postmodern approaches have now become sufficiently widespread that their practitioners should engage in a constructive self-critique if they are to avoid promoting a new orthodoxy. In other words, postmodern practice, like the traditional approaches it critiques, can *also* unfold along colonial dynamics. Even our emancipatory ideals can be turned into unilateral relationships that defy the spirit of collaboration. We are aware of this dynamic occurring at times in our own work, and we witness it in the work of our colleagues. In this book, we willingly turn the mirror on ourselves and propose ways of preventing our cherished theories and epistemologies from swallowing the persons who consult us. The hope here is to cultivate what Derrida (2001) describes as "an ethic of hospitality" (p. 16) to the other, an openness to all points of view and an exchange among diverse ways of knowing that is not mutually exclusive but "both/and" or "one and the other at the same time."

REFERENCES

Bruner, J. (1987). Life as narrative. *Social Research 54*(1):12-32.

Caputo, J.D. (Ed.) (1997). *Deconstruction in a Nutshell: A Conversation with Jacques Derrida.* New York: Fordham University Press.

Cornell, D. (1992). *The Philosophy of the Limit.* New York and London: Routledge.

Derrida, J. (2001). *Cosmopolitanism and Forgiveness: Thinking in Action.* London: Routledge.

Foucault, M. (1980). *Power/Knowledge: Selected Interviews and Other Writings.* New York: Pantheon.

Gergen, K. (1999). *An Invitation to Social Construction.* Thousand Oaks, CA: Sage.

Habermas, J. (1972). *Knowledge and Human Interests.* Boston: Beacon Press.

Larner, G. (1999). Derrida and the deconstruction of power as context and topic in therapy. In I. Parker (Ed.) *Deconstructing Psychotherapy* (pp. 39-53). London: Sage.

Lyotard, J.F. (1984). *The Postmodern Condition: A Report on Knowledge.* Minneapolis: University of Minnesota Press.

Paré, D.A. (1999). Towards a place to stand: The meeting of discourses in counselor education. In *Conference Proceedings of New Zealand Association of Counselors Annual Conference* (pp. 88-95). Hamilton, New Zealand: New Zealand Association of Counsellors.

Paré, D.A. (2001). Finding a place to stand: Reflections on discourse and intertextuality in counseling practice. In J.R. Morss, N. Stephenson, and H. van Rappard (Eds.), *Theoretical Issues in Psychology: Proceedings of the International Society for Theoretical Psychology 1999 Conference* (pp. 327-339). Norwell, MA: Kluwer Academic Publishers.

Polkinghorne, D. (1993). Postmodern epistemology of practice. In S. Kvale (Ed.), *Psychology and Postmodernism* (pp. 147-165). Newbury Park, CA: Sage.

Rorty, R. (1979). *Philosophy and the Mirror of Nature*. Princeton, NJ: Princeton University Press.

Shotter, J. (1993). *The Cultural Politics of Everyday Life*. Buckingham, UK: Open University Press.

Todd, N. and Wade, A. (1994). Domination, deficiency, and psychotherapy. Part I. *The Calgary Participator* 4(1):37-46.

Weber, S. (1987). *Institution and Interpretation*. Minneapolis: University of Minnesota Press.

THEORY:
BEYOND PERSUASION—
THEORIZING WITHOUT VIOLENCE

Chapter 1

Social Construction As Practical Theory: Lessons for Practice and Reflection in Psychotherapy

Sheila McNamee

Theory constructs the world. One need only look as far as Karl Marx's analysis of class struggle or Adam Smith's ideas on free market economies to see how theory moves nations and shapes history. There clearly is much that is generative in theory and much that is destructive. Sheila McNamee is sensitized to the potential violence of ideas and also to the manner in which the meaning of an idea is coconstituted by speaker and listener, as she communicates about social constructionism. The apparently simple act of writing about theory is rendered far more complex, and potentially hazardous, when one considers that the meaning that emerges is a function of both writer and reader.

This chapter provides an alternative to well-established traditions of persuasion, defying the usual convention of laying out the boundaries of a theory. In effect, it is more an invitation than a "telling." McNamee seeks here not to convince readers of her point of view so much as provide an opportunity to glimpse and reflect on ideas associated with social constructionism. A central theme is the inescapable link between idea and practice. Social constructionism directs us not to "who we are," but rather encourages a mindfulness about the active, ongoing, relational process of meaning making.

Much has been written on social construction, relational realities, and the implications of these views in psychology and psychotherapeutic practice. And although many of us have devoted a good deal of time and effort to connecting theory and practice, there remains an overwhelming frustration about what we *do* differently when we operate from a constructionist sensibility. That sensibility leads us to view social constructionism not so much as a theory that proposes particular techniques or methods for practice, but rather something more akin to a relational practice, a way of making sense of and engaging with the world that invites others into dialogue. This emphasis on the ongoing coconstruction of meaning renders incomplete any categorical statements about what social constructionist practice "is" or "is not" because it excludes the response of those with whom these statements are shared: calling specific therapeutic practices more relational than individualist is, itself, a situated, relational activity.

Central to this chapter is the intriguing dilemma of articulating theory and practice in a manner that is closer to an invitation to dialogue than a closed pronouncement of how things are. The dilemma hinges on the notion that becoming a proponent of certain theories and practices has less to do with achieving the proper skill and more to do with embracing a particular vocabulary for action. Our working vocabulary for action—the manner in which we engage with others in the production of meaning—speaks more to the tenor of our practice than do any specific techniques or methods. The vocabulary for action is the focus of this contribution.

We repeatedly hear that there is no constructionist method per se. Constructionism itself does not dictate specific techniques or methods. Yet, as a practical theory (Shotter, 1993; Gergen, 1999), constructionism informs us in our activities, both at the level of theoretical talk and at the level of professional and everyday practices. The challenge, then, is of articulating a constructionist sensibility—a sensibility intent on the relational aspects of meaning, including theoretical meaning—while avoiding the creation of a tightly conscripted set of techniques or procedures. My hope is that in attempting to do this here I will help to illuminate what is distinctive about social constructionism. Rather than an explanatory narrative about therapeutic change or human nature, social constructionism is a theory about *meaning* and, more particularly, about meaning as a relational practice. Rather than prescribing certain specific therapeutic interventions, it encourages us to reflect upon what sorts of relationship practices various therapeutic theories invite us to employ. Social constructionism is, then, a theory *about* theories, and one that reminds us that theories ultimately are relational practices.

This poses some intriguing questions about presenting social constructionism. Is it possible to engage others *relationally* through sharing constructionist ideas without formally listing or prescribing how to "be" relational? Is there a way to passionately embrace constructionism without it becoming dogma or absolute truth? Do the discussions about it need to be formed in opposition to other, already well-developed orientations (e.g., individualism)? Is there a way to talk about social construction without alienating other discursive forms? These questions hinge on a central distinction between talk as rhetoric and persuasion versus talk as overture.

PERSUASION AS PERVASIVE

Persuasion, as a cultural resource, has a powerful history and a powerful effect on our everyday activities. The discussion of persuasion is traced to Aristotle. In Aristotle's *Rhetoric and Poetics,* he argues that rhetoric is the ability to find the available means of persuasion in a situation (1954, p. 24). He proceeds to articulate the most effective means of influencing others (i.e., persuading others), which hinge on notions of rationality or logic. His perspective was guided by his belief that truth is gained by opposition and the means by which to oppose another is via formal logic.

Obviously Aristotle's work has been influential. It remains a mainstay of cultural discussion and everyday practice. Debate, a common form of public discourse in our culture, is rooted in Aristotelian logic. Debate is centered on influencing others—winning an argument through influence or persuasion, that is, through logic or rationality. But the question is, *which* logic or rationality? And who gets to decide which logic or rationality? We are hard-pressed to find situations in which our conversations do not take the form of persuading another to accept or buy our argument.

As an illustration, I recently had an interesting conversation with a colleague. He teaches courses in argumentation informed by classical rhetoric. I teach courses in dialogue processes informed by social construction. The meeting evolved into a discussion of some longstanding issues in our department, and the challenge we faced was to proceed in a manner that promoted constructive mutual dialogue on the topic. My colleague, the expert in argumentation, claimed that when we discuss things as a department we need to start with the *facts* and from there our job is to persuade one another by bringing evidence to the fore. Whichever argument succeeds dictates how we go on together. I questioned his claim by asking, "But whose facts? Facts by what standards? And what would count as evidence?" The answer: *"The* facts. *The* evidence." Well, I wondered out loud, isn't it the case that what counts as a fact is what is constructed in activity (language) with others? Thus, when any subgroup in the department gathers "evidence" on an issue, it is in the process of *creating* a fact, *creating* evidence, and thus *creating* what will count as good, as bad, as right, and as wrong. Incommensurate beliefs emerge within one small academic department. If we consider that everyone is potentially creating a different rationality, could we use this recognition to *begin* our conversations from a stance of curiosity or interested inquiry? Might we not come to the table with genuine questions about what counts as a fact or as evidence to each person? If we did that, how might our "deliberations" be different?

Frustrated, my colleague informed me that the world operates within an argumentative model. We persuade. It is the judgment made by the group concerning the quality and validity of the argument (based on the facts and the evidence) that determines the course of action. To him, discussion of what will count as a fact would detract from efficiency and prevent us from moving forward as a group. (As someone who consults to organizations, I hear this critique of dialogue quite often.) In the spirit of multivocality, of embracing multiple viewpoints, I chose not to attempt to refute my colleague's assessment. I did, however, invite him to consider the potential efficiency of spending a good chunk of time every once in a while clarifying the various beliefs, meanings, values, and so forth of group members because the time taken to do this might help to establish relationships that recognize and value difference rather than relationships that either deny or exaggerate difference. Once appreciative relationships are established, members have additional resources available for connecting with one another, for understanding how others might respond or operate in a particular moment. The mutual exploration of values, commitments, moralities—as well as the relational communities which give the values, commitments, and moralities sustenance—can offer provocations for future engagement. In effect, my response was an overture to dialogue, to a mode of meaning making, founded on a mutual going forward, a collaboration rather than a rivalry.

PROVIDING A CONVERSATIONAL ARENA

It is by now probably obvious that persuading the reader to "buy" my argument for social construction and relational practices is a job I do not wish to take on here—a job not in keeping with the constructionist premises that inform my work and this chapter. The main premise of social construction is that meaning is not an individual phenomenon. It is not located in the private mind of a person, nor is it unilaterally determined by one person. Meaning (and thus reality), to the constructionist, is an achievement of people coordinating their activities together. I believe my colleagues and I might have more success "going on together" if we approach issues as challenges in co-construction rather than as facts to be contested and countered. We might not always agree on the meaning of an action, a situation, or a relationship, but whatever meaning we construct is always an emergent by-product of what we do together. Thus, one person alone cannot control the outcome of any conversation, relationship, or situation—and therein lies the intriguing challenge of this chapter. To convey theory is to make meaning, and I cannot make meaning alone. How you take in my words is as critical to what this conversation produces as the words I commit to paper. I cannot prevent you from reading this chapter as propaganda or persuasive rhetoric designed to convert you to social constructionism. All I can do is attempt to provide a *conversational arena* where multiple logics, coherences, realities can be coordinated.

From the story about my conversation with my colleague, I think you may appreciate how institutional life, and indeed the wider society, tends to operate on the principle that "good arguments" begin with "good facts" and "good evidence." But whose definition of "good" are we using? This is the question that often, when handled in an adversarial manner or when posed as a debate, can fracture and divide relationships. This is not to suggest debate and argument are "wrong"; it is only to say that there are always limits to the utility of any way of acting. Not only is it difficult to be sensitive to the multiplicity of moralities and beliefs in any community, but it is difficult to forge new ways of relating that value such multiplicity. At this moment, you and I are confronted with the same limitations. How can text, which once published remains unaltered, invite many voices and possibilities and not be read as the "truth" or the "facts" or the "evidence"? My hope is that by sharing the conversations within which many of these issues arise for me, by writing in a mode that might be viewed more as an invitation into conversation than as an authoritative voice, we might together approach an ongoing conversation in which multiple possibilities can emerge. Toward that end, I invite you to view this offering, and others like it, as openings, invitations, challenges, or proposals into new ways of relating together.

I will therefore refrain from saying that social construction is the answer to the world's problems or telling you that a certain set of practices illustrates social construction in action and others do not. I will instead try to address the question of what we mean by the term *social construction,* why many refer to social construction as a generative or practical theory, and what difference this might make in our day-to-day lives.

SOCIAL CONSTRUCTION

When someone asks me what I mean by using the term *social construction* I feel a rush of anxiety. I wonder how to describe social construction without having my conversational partner either glaze over in a sea of abstraction or nod enthusiastically saying, "Oh yes, that's just common sense. You mean being open-minded."

It is precisely this problem of meaning that is the central issue of social construction. For the social constructionist, meaning does not reside within individuals, requiring competent or accurate communication to convey one's meanings to another. I am not holding the correct interpretation of social construction and using my words here to convey my meaning to you. Rather, I am attempting to use terms that invite us all to generate new resources for action, new ways of making sense that will support us in our actions. My hope is that my words serve as openings to new understandings, to confirmation of understandings we might already carry, to provocations, to questions, to a wider range of possibilities. Meaning is created in the coordination of activities among people. To that end, the meaning of social construction is *actively* coordinated by *us* in our ongoing activities— including the writing and reading of this chapter. At this very moment, you and I are engaged in an active process of coordination. Later, as you converse with others who have read these words, the meaning of those very words has the potential to change and shift all the more. Meaning is never fixed. It is not stable and unchanging. There is, then, no way for me, *once and for all,* to tell you what I mean. My colleague, John Shotter, captures the indeterminacy of meaning whenever someone asks him what he means. He responds, "I don't know. We haven't finished talking yet!" No meaning is fixed for all time. We often operate on the principle that we have "settled the issue once and for all," but new conversations, new relationships, new situations will continue to transform meaning.

Film director Arthur Penn recently offered me a beautiful illustration of this point. He was talking about his film, *Little Big Man* (1970) starring Dustin Hoffman. In the story, Dustin Hoffman's character is accepted, as a white man, into a Native American tribe. In fact, he is allowed to marry into the tribe. After a bloody battle leaving the tribe depleted of its males, Hoffman's pregnant wife—a member of the tribe—asks him to engage in sexual encounters with her sisters in hope of impregnating them and thereby ensuring the continuation of the tribe. An action that would otherwise be considered immoral and certainly inappropriate to this community is now transformed into a positive and necessary action. As Penn describes it, "As conditions change through (in this case) tragedy, we see that values, language, and morality change as well. It is the elasticity of meaning that is important to recognize and this, to me, is what social construction is about" (personal communication, May 2001). I think that Arthur Penn has beautifully captured this relational appreciation for meaning. It shifts not willy-nilly to suit one's needs but rather cautiously and curiously to address the complexities of life.

Reorienting ourselves away from a view that meaning is in our heads requires a significant shift, and it is a difficult shift to make. The next section discusses this issue, phrasing it in terms that invite some new conversations to take place among us.

MEANING AS RELATIONAL

It seems only natural to us to accept the idea that meaning is an individual's possession. After all, when I look around, I see bodies that are separate from my own and from others. I see eyes that are yours, hands that are yours, gestures that belong to you, and even peculiar phrasings, intonations, and quirky movements that *are* you. Who would want to question whether you have private thoughts, ideas, motivations, intentions, aspirations, emotions, and more? Is it not the wide variation among our private motivations, intentions, ideas, and so forth that makes living so difficult? Are not all the problems of the world, of social life, linked to the problem of meaning? Poor performance in school is a sign of a student's inability to grasp the correct meaning of the material. Social injustices, such as prejudice, are easily explained as the by-products of those who do not "understand" what is good and what is bad, what is right and what is wrong. Genocide, economic instability, religious oppression would cease to exist if we could control meaning.

The problem is that we cannot control meaning. By locating meaning within individual minds, we contribute to the complexity of the problem. If only we could design the *right* therapeutic technique, we could eradicate depression. If we could create pedagogical practices that work for particular topics or types of people, we could educate the masses. These hopes are heavily layered with that sense of rationality and logic which we inherit from the influence of science in our culture. There is a simple method that will lead us to truth—not only to truth but to truth with assurance.

Just as the portrayal here of meaning as relational represents a discourse that invites certain ways of thinking and acting, so does the portrayal of meaning as residing within individuals. This latter discourse has a very long history, and is exceedingly pervasive within the institution of psychology. It is manifest in the belief that professionals know what it means to be psychologically healthy and are able to recognize signs of mental instability through the actions of clients. It proposes that years of experience on the part of professionals yield effective therapeutic practices and correct diagnoses.

When we entertain a relational view of meaning, these premises take on a very different light. If we talk about meaning as a by-product of our coordinations—our joint actions—with others, then what is the job of the therapist? More generally, what does the field of psychology, from this relational orientation, offer? Social construction, with its relational focus, presents a challenge to traditional notions of expert knowledge and professional neutrality.

If meaning is constructed in the joint activities of persons in relation, then any theory or model is not a truth telling but a very *local* way of understanding. It is local in that it is produced in relation to others in the immediate circumstances (even if they are only virtually connected). The "telling" that this chapter represents is an example of just this: in the local junction between you as reader and me as writer, meaning is constructed, to be taken forward to other encounters with other persons at other times and in other places. That meaning is inevitably a function of the cultural traditions, local conventions, historical canons, and so forth that speak through our tongues and hear through our ears. This view leads us away from the mutual trumping that accompanies a competitive quest for the truth. Instead, we are faced with the question of how to live together in a complex world inhabited by so many differing beliefs, truths, values, and so forth. The task at hand is one of coordination, and our curiosity is drawn to therapy as a site of coordinated meaning making.

FROM METHOD TO DAILY ENGAGEMENTS (PERFORMANCES)

On a broader scale, the discourse of science as the privileged and trustworthy approach to *discovering* knowledge, truth, and (perhaps most important) solutions still permeates the culture at large. We need only go to our local bookstores and glance at the recent bestsellers. Titles promising simple steps to remedy families, marriages, businesses, neighborhoods, and organizations are profuse. Add to this the bind many of us confront when we attempt to argue for the "legitimacy" of our work within the boundaries of traditional scientific discourse. If we dismiss (i.e., refuse to acknowledge) the criteria of scientific discourse—of modernism—as the ultimate and pure form of legitimation, we are very quickly disregarded. It is worth noting that many graduate students and young professionals interested in postmodern discourse feel frustrated by the oppressive demands placed upon them by those championing the individualist tradition. I believe the frustration and failure to open generative dialogue with those who are more traditional in their orientation has little to do with the traditionalists' lack of interest in or respect for such dialogue. Rather, I believe the frustration and failure that emerges from these conversations is couched in the confrontational and accusatory approach that often accompanies such dialogues. The very same approach that those of us attracted to postmodern discourse (and social construction) find limiting (i.e., the debate format in which one truth oppresses another—all couched in that old tradition of persuasion) is unfortunately used to argue in favor of postmodernism. In the language of Watzlawick, Weakland, and Fisch (1974), postmodernists attempting to champion the case for postmodernism by arguing *against* modernism as a first-order change—simply substituting one action with another similar action thereby maintaining the pattern rather than changing it. Now, instead of modernism with its focus on individualism being "true," postmodernism with its focus on the relational construction of meaning is true. The actual point of postmodernism is that neither is true in the traditional sense. Both are *discursive options* and to put it this way is to achieve, I think, second-order change (change of the argument entirely).

It may appear that I am proposing we give up the dominant individualist (scientific, modernist) discourse. I am not. Instead, I propose we augment the individualist discourse with an alternative discourse—in this case, the relational discourse proposed within a constructionist sensibility. Would not a conversation be inviting if it were not claiming that individualism is inherently wrong or bad? The job we have as social constructionists is to invite ourselves and others into conversations that allow all voices to be heard. To remain open to a multiplicity of views on practice is not to offer a blanket endorsement, and it also is not to selectively dismiss. By not being dismissive, we continue to construct meaning together, making it possible to keep the conversation going.

When we refigure meaning as relational, we regard it as a practice, a *performance* that inevitably involves more than one participant. This draws our attention to the *process* of meaning making as well as the *relationship* within which meaning is constructed. We are less focused on the "proper" or "best" way to be professionals or provide information. Our focus, instead, is centered on the multiple ways in which social transformation can take place. Further, our focus is centered on the participants engaged in the immediate moment and the wide array of both common and diverse voices, relations, communities, and experiences that each brings to the current context.

SOCIAL CONSTRUCTION AS PRACTICAL THEORY

As theorists and practitioners we have choices about how to use the theories that inform our work. We can approach theories and perspectives, be they individualist or relational, as telling us the "truth" about the way the social world operates. On the other hand, we can ask ourselves when it might be useful to draw on resources offered by one theory or approach as opposed to another. To ask this question requires a sensitivity to the interactive moment, to the historical and cultural conditions that construct our worlds, and to the multiple voices that participate in shaping who we are and what we are doing. Social constructionism encourages us to consider how any particular idea or discourse converts to practice in the performance of a *specific moment* in relationship with another—rather than turning to a canonical truth that prescribes Theory A or Model B.

I hope that this very brief description of social construction is not read as yet another truth telling. Social construction, like any other theory, is a form of coordinated activity among persons in relation. To that end, every theory is about practice. We need to spend more time, I think, asking what sorts of practices are invited by the different stories each theory tells. I have tried to sketch the ways in which social construction could offer a set of fluid resources for action that do not eliminate or demonize other traditions. Those of us who adopt social construction are not attempting to claim a preferred mode of life or to discover the best way for a person, a relationship, an organization, or a community to develop. Social construction, instead, urges us to attend to the traditions, the communities, the situated practices of the participants at hand (i.e., to local understandings) in identifying what becomes real, true, and good. To attend to traditions, communities, and situated practices requires a constant flexibility on the part of those involved. Where the purpose of modernist theory and practice is to solve problems, cure illness, and achieve social, environmental, and scientific advancement, the purpose of social construction, as a discursive option, is to explore what sorts of social life become possible when one way of talking and acting is employed versus another. The alternative that social construction offers is a relational discourse—one that views meaningful action as always emerging within relationship (whether those relationships are "real," imagined, or virtual). The purpose is not to determine whether the modernist focus on individualism or the postmodern focus on the relational should dominate.

The metaphor of meaning as performance is useful because it makes a ritualized practice familiar. It cuts meaning from a focus on methods for conveying knowledge to a process which is attentive to the ways in which participants create meaning together. As we engage with one another in therapy we create not only a sense of who we are but also a sense of what is valued. We create—perform *together*—a world, a lived reality.

The metaphor of performance provides the opportunity for us to engage in self-reflexive inquiry about our own resources for action which are not being utilized but which might aid in creating ways of going on together (see McNamee and Gergen, 1998). If meaning is a by-product of relational engagement (conversation, performance), then we are free to pause and ask ourselves what other ways might we talk about this topic, this issue, this problem. Performance as a metaphor enhances self-reflexivity by legitimizing it. In so doing, we open ourselves to listening, reading, talking, and writing in more "generous" modes—remaining open to the relational coherence of diverse ways of acting. We thereby avoid speaking with a sense of certainty that the world is or should be one way. In so doing we open possibilities for the coordination of multiple ways of being human and of, as Wittgenstein (1953) says, "going on together."

REFERENCES

Aristotle (R. McKeon, Ed.) (1954). *Rhetoric and poetics.* New York: Modern Library.

Gergen, K.J. (1999). *An invitation to social construction.* London: Sage Publications.

McNamee, S. and Gergen, K.J. (1998). *Relational responsibility: Resources for sustainable dialogue.* Thousand Oaks, CA: Sage Publications.

Shotter, J. (1993). *Conversational realities.* London: Sage Publications.

Watzlawick, P., Weakland, J., and Fisch, R. (1974). *Change: Principles of problem formation and problem resolution.* New York: W.W. Norton.

Wittgenstein, L. (1953). *Philosophical investigations.* Translated by G. Anscombe. New York: Macmillan.

SUGGESTED READINGS

Gergen, K.J. (1999). *An invitation to social construction.* London: Sage Publications.

Holzman, L. (Ed.) (1999). *Performing psychology: A postmodern culture of the mind.* New York: Routledge.

McNamee, S. and Gergen, K.J. (1998). *Relational responsibility: Resources for sustainable dialogue.* Thousand Oaks, CA: Sage Publications.

Chapter 2

Therapy Theory
After the Postmodern Turn

Lois Shawver

There is a certain comfort that accompanies an expert stance, a reassurance that comes with adopting a position of certainty. The notion that we have unlocked the code of human nature, or the therapeutic change process, helps to justify interventions and mutes the nagging voice of self-doubt. In this chapter, Lois Shawver describes the disenchantment experienced by many within psychology in the wake of the so-called Dodo Bird Verdict, the conclusion of research indicating that all therapies seem to be about equally helpful. For many, this was the end of a modern hope for therapy designed around the scientist practitioner model. If we cannot speak definitively about which approaches work for which complaints, how do we legitimize ourselves, why should anyone consult us, and how should we proceed? Shawver's response to the Dodo Bird Verdict is an alternate vision of the work. Paralogy—a term initially coined by Jean-François Lyotard—embraces dialogue, and a form of talk oriented more to listening than talking.

For a long time, therapists pinned their hopes for a better therapy on the dream that one day therapy practice would be grounded in scientific research. When that day came, so everyone hoped, the therapist could decide what to do in therapy simply by looking at the data and seeing what worked, or even what correct beliefs could be passed on to clients in the form of advice (e.g., Glover, 1926; Harms, 1970; Karpman, 1947; Ornstein, 1968; Maultsby, 1968; Thorne, 1953). Only then, so the dream told them, would therapists be able to escape superstition and bias and become "scientific-practitioners" (Raimy, 1950).

I have come to think of this scientific practitioner model of therapy as the *modern hope* and to contrast it with the *postmodern hope* that now inspires me. Although the modern hope is still very much alive in academic circles (O'Sullivan and Quevillon, 1992; Peterson, 2000), therapists in the field today are often disillusioned with it (Klein, 1995; Martin, 1995; Rennie, 1994; Stiles, 1995; Lionell, 2000; Young and Heller, 2000; Robinson, 2000; Schwartz, 2000).

There is a story behind this disillusionment. When the modern hope was still an untarnished dream, research projects were launched far and wide in order to ground psychotherapy in science. At first these studies seemed mildly encouraging, but then researchers began taking a closer look. On this closer look it seemed to be simply impossible to decide which kind of therapy, or which technique or advice, was most supported by research. In fact, all therapies seemed to be about equally effective, and some research even suggested that all therapies were about equally effective as no therapy at all (Eysenck 1952, 1966; Lambert and Bergin, 1994). This hit at the heart of the modern dream for therapists to someday become scientific practitioners.

These discouraging findings were first announced in a publication by Luborsky, Singer, and Luborsky (1975). They announced their conclusion by calling it the "Dodo Bird Verdict." It's a catchy metaphor. The dodo bird in *Alice's Adventures in Wonderland* (Carroll, 1946) declared that all the competitors in a foot race were winners because each had run in a different direction. The analogy was that therapy researchers, much like the racers in Wonderland, defined their individual goals so differently that there was no way to compare therapies. Research was not able to decide which kind of therapy worked better, or which kind of therapy to use with which client (Luborsky, 1995; Wampold et al., 1997), and this kind of differential seemed essential for the modern hope of therapists becoming scientific practitioners.

As Martin Seligman (1995) wrote, the Dodo Bird Verdict came "as a rude shock to efficacy researchers [studying therapy], since the main theme of efficacy studies [had] been the demonstration of the usefulness of specific techniques for specific disorders" (p. 969). This Seligman article was published in *American Psychologist*. In writing this article, Seligman, I feel, had his finger on the pulse of the clinician who was growing increasingly impatient with research that felt irrelevant and empty. It is noteworthy that three years after this publication, Martin Seligman was elected president of the American Psychological Association.

For many of us, the Dodo Bird Verdict simply burst our balloons. Next, we stopped identifying with one school or another (since none could be proven better by research) and began calling ourselves eclectic (Jensen, Bergin, and Greaves, 1990). It was then that the disappointed therapists began to ask: What should we do? Many thought: We can no longer justify acting like experts in therapy process and in human affairs. What do we do now?

Hynan (1981) suggested we do whatever we want to do, since it did not seem to matter much what we did. But many of us were not ready to say that "anything goes" (Chessick, 1995; Phillips, 1998; Smith, 1991; Shawver, 1983; Shotter, 1992; Strenger and Omer, 1992). After all, if one says "anything goes" then this would seem to open the door to exploitation and abuse.

But if not "anything goes," then how *should* we do therapy? Without a scientific grounding, how could we be anything more than advocates for our personal belief systems or biases? It was quite a dilemma.

Then, thank goodness, came the postmodern literature with its new *postmodern hope* for assisting with this sticky problem by providing a kind of therapy less dependent on a scientific foundation. The emergence of this postmodern eclecticism did not go unnoticed (Larsen, 1999).

OUR POSTMODERN TURN

Still, I do admit that it can take an experienced therapist a moment to recognize the promise of a postmodern therapy. All postmodern philosophy is not equally hopeful. In fact, much postmodern thinking seems nihilistic and despairing.

But do not let that confuse you. Even when "postmodern" was an embryonic concept in a few obscure books, it had already polarized into two main types, one negative and skeptical and one affirmative and hopeful. Thus, early on, Rosenberg and White (1957) said postmodernism was something to celebrate, and Irving Howe (1959) and Harry Levin (1960) called it as something to deplore. Later, when

Ihab Hassan (1970) applauded postmodernism, Leslie Fiedler (1971, pp. 379-400) energetically denounced it.

It was Pauline Rosenau (1992) who put it all in perspective when she said that the two poles of postmodernism were so different that we could really speak of two postmodernisms. She labeled these "skeptical" and "affirmative," and here is how she distinguished them:

> The skeptical post-modernism (or merely skeptics), offering a pessimistic, negative, gloomy assessment, argue that the postmodern age is one of fragmentation, disintegration, malaise, meaninglessness, a vagueness or even absence of moral parameters and social chaos. (p. 15)

In contrast, she explained, "affirmative postmodernism" is

> a more hopeful, optimistic view of the post-modern age . . . Most affirmative postmoderns seek a philosophical and ontological intellectual practice that is nondogmatic, tentative, and nonideological . . . (pp. 15-16)

Defined in this way, skeptical postmoderns today might include Baudrillard (1983), Cushman (1990), Cushman and Gilford (1999), and Glass (1993) while affirmative postmoderns would include Lyotard (1979, 1984), Rorty (1979), Gergen (1995), McNamee and Gergen (1992), Anderson (1997), Newman and Holzman (1996, 1997), Shotter (1992), Hoffman (2001), Andersen (1991), and, I would argue, most important, a certain reading of Ludwig Wittgenstein (1963).

Let me be more specific. Along with Lynn Hoffman (2001), as well as John Walter and Jane Peller (2000, p. 15), I am inclined to think of Michael White and Steve de Shazer as more poststructuralist rather than postmodern. There are different ways to define postmodernism, but this is the classification scheme that I believe causes the least confusion: Poststructuralists in therapy theory tend to be more inspired by Foucault's writing and the hope of revisioning historical accounts or narratives (i.e., "genealogies") that are more true than the traditional and popular accounts. The affirmative postmoderns, however, tend to be inspired by later Wittgenstein and/or Lyotard, and their postmodern approaches are relatively open textured. They may advocate ways of creating more generative conversation but they do not do much to control the content of the emerging conversation. Postmodern approaches look for new ways to talk that create new conversational paths and new solutions to particular, and typically situational, problems.

Back to my story. When the Dodo Bird Verdict came down, many therapists became skeptical that science could really help them become scientific practitioners. This meant that these disillusioned therapists, often without realizing it, became skeptical postmoderns. But as time went on a new promise emerged. It was a new affirmative postmodernism. Some of the skeptical postmoderns feel the inspiration. As Lyotard (1984, p. 81) writes, there is a group of us talking today who are no longer nostalgic about the lost modern hope because something new and exciting is opening up before us.

THE NEW VISION OF AFFIRMATIVE POSTMODERNISM

What is this new affirmative postmodern promise? To my way of thinking, it is a new kind of conversation. My favorite word for it is *paralogy,* after the famous postmodern philosopher Jean-François Lyotard (1984). It is a special kind of conversation happening in postmodern circles and it is, I believe, a good answer to therapy theory's Dodo Bird Verdict, at least for now.

But before I explain what paralogy is, let me ask you to keep your ear tuned to hearing the word *modern* as something other than "up to date." In the postmodern literature, modern has come to mean something more like "pretends to be more scientific that it really is." *Modern* conversation tends toward "dispute" because the facts are not empirically established but each side's claims are right. Postmodern conversation tends toward paralogy.

So what is paralogy? Paralogy is a kind of conversation in which people rethink things, partly by rearranging what they already know (Wittgenstein, 1963, p. 109), and partly by fostering more creative imagination (Lyotard, 1984, p. 52) for solving specific and often local problems.

Perhaps a few sample illustrations will be helpful. Let us look first at a model of *modern conversation.* In its simplest form a modern conversation might go like this:

PAT: The central thing everybody needs to be happy is self-esteem.

KIM: Not so. The central thing everybody needs is love.

PAT: I have read X and he says that it is self-esteem we need.

KIM: Well, X is wrong. Look here. Y says it is love that is required.

Kim could also be modern by endorsing Pat's claim so that there was no revision of the initial theories, no creative theorizing. But in either case, the underlying modern (or scientistic) idea is that if one theory wins, the other loses.

In contrast, here is an illustration of postmodern conversation, or paralogy. Notice how the different theories evolve in collaboration as long as the conversation continues:

PAT: The central thing everybody needs to be happy is self-esteem.

KIM: Well, yes, but love is important, too.

PAT: I think self-esteem must come first. People won't love you if you don't love yourself first.

KIM: For me, love comes first. If I have that, then my self-esteem is sky high.

PAT: I can remember a romantic relationship that made me feel that way, sent my self-esteem to the sky.

KIM: So, love comes first for you, too?

PAT: Maybe not. I think the self-esteem was really false and made me vulnerable when he left me.

Both Pat and Kim are postmodern and paralogical in their conversation. Can you see how Pat's story changed without her mimicking Kim's story? And how Kim listened and was able to present a different point of view without claiming that her view told the whole story? It is this change and evolution in the story that marks paralogy.

Now, I want to contrast modern and postmodern conversation as they might be enacted in therapy sessions. In a *modern* session, we might hear the therapist telling the client what the problem is, and perhaps disputing with the client about it:

CLIENT: My problem is I need more self-esteem.

THERAPIST: What you really need is to speak up for yourself.

CLIENT: If I had more self-esteem, maybe I could.

THERAPIST: Just learn to speak up for yourself. That must come first. Self-esteem comes later.

Can you see how a modern therapist would need research to lend legitimacy to such an authoritative stance? It is possible, however, for the conversation to sound far less authoritarian and still be modern in my view, so let me give you a sample of that. I consider the following to be modern because there is no ongoing rearrangement of the information, no restructuring in improvisational process.

CLIENT: My problem is I need more self-esteem.
THERAPIST: Would that help you?
CLIENT: If I had more self-esteem, I'd be a lot more successful.
THERAPIST: Why don't you have more self-esteem?

Here the therapist is not a collaborator in the creation of new meaning with new twists and paths in the accounts of things. Instead, the therapist stays entirely within the client's frame.

In contrast, paralogy is a way of conversing that allows new ideas to emerge (Lyotard, 1984, p. 61). Everything in the previous conversation takes place within the same point of view. Still, the conversation at least avoids the authoritarian stance that is so inappropriate in our postmodern era, and it is even possible that the conversation will take a postmodern turn. For example, imagine the dialogue taking the following turn:

PATIENT: [laughing] I don't have enough self-esteem to say.
THERAPIST: Do you have enough courage to guess?

Here I would say the therapist becomes more postmodern by introducing the new concept (i.e., "courage") without disputing the old one (i.e., "self-esteem").

Let me give you an example of what I would consider therapeutic paralogy. Here both therapist and client contribute ideas and associations to the conversation yet neither defends a position and there is some real paralogical rearrangement of ideas between them. Neither comes away with the same old story. Notice also how the dialogue stays close to specifics. I believe specifics help bring out the paralogy.

CLIENT: I just need more self-esteem.

THERAPIST: Why do you say that?

CLIENT: Well, like at work. Others go to lunch but I just work right through it even though I'm really way ahead of all the rest.

THERAPIST: You sound industrious.

CLIENT: Yes, I guess so—but at the same time I'm envious of the others having fun. I wish I could be lazy like that, too.

THERAPIST: Lazy? Yesterday you said your dad was lazy. Is that how you want to be?

CLIENT: I don't want to be that lazy!

THERAPIST: Just a little more lazy, just at lunch time?

CLIENT: Just thinking of Dad makes me want to work through lunch [laughs].

THERAPIST: Which would be OK, but you also said you felt envious that the guys were going out.

CLIENT: Well, there's that, too.

At this point, the therapist has already introduced ideas and associations, but notice, as the conversation continues, how the therapist introduces still another idea that inspires the client's imagination and in turn sparks another idea in the client, different from the one that the therapist had. Now, picture the following as a conversation continuing from the previous excerpt.

THERAPIST: You know, when I think about it, you don't reject *everything* about your dad. You admire his way of making friends.

CLIENT: I do admire that, but maybe I'm afraid if I tried to copy that I'd turn out to be a bum like him.

See how it was agreed that the client admired his dad? But in the process of agreeing, the client generated still a different idea, the idea of the client being afraid of turning out to be a bum. Agreement exists at times in the conversation but only as states in the conversational process (Lyotard, 1984, p. 65). Similarly, disagreement is also just a stage and does not become dispute. In paralogy, agreement is not particularly valued in and of itself. The point is to generate interesting ideas that make sense in the conversational quest of paralogy (Lyotard, 1984, p. 60).

At least as I see it, in such a paralogical therapy the therapist contributes substantively to the dialogue, introducing new words and metaphors that can reframe things without demeaning alternate frames. The old model of therapist as expert gives way to the model of therapist who fosters new conversational paths without insisting on any of them. Each frame opens new conversational paths that were not foreseen by client or therapist.

If therapy works paralogically, then for a postmodern mind there seems no reason for one form of therapy to trump another with definitive research. The therapy *is* the research—research that never knows the answer for sure and forever, but finds workable solutions for presenting problems. Each solution succeeds or fails on its own terms in its own context, not in a competitive race against others. As Lyotard put it, paralogy is not a zero-sum game (Lyotard, 1984, p. 67). To return to the disillusioning Dodo Bird Verdict, all kinds of therapies can be winners (or losers). We must feel our way through somewhat unknown paths in hopes of finding success for each problem or each client. And although the final results are never certain, something is valuable, at least, in the client pooling intelligence with another human (the therapist) to do what seems best in the moment.

Although paralogy is a word that I prefer for this kind of conversation, others seem to call the same thing something else. It seems to me, for example, that Tom Andersen's (1991) reflecting teams work paralogically, as does Harlene Anderson's (1997) style of therapeutic conversation. It is what Sheila McNamee (in Chapter 1, p. 11) calls providing a "*conversational arena* where multiple logics, coherences, realities can be coordinated." Lynn Hoffman (2001) seems to be looking for paralogical ways for us to collaborate conversationally with our clients, as are Sheila McNamee and Ken Gergen (1992) and many others. I believe such conversation is at the heart of new affirmative postmodernism in psychotherapy theory and the possibility that we can do this kind of therapy without waiting for research to ground our practice represents a postmodern hope—the postmodern hope, in fact, that inspires me.

CREATING PARALOGY

This takes us to the question of how to create paralogy, how to keep therapy conversation from deteriorating into a modern dispute. As a paralogist, I will not give you a final formula, but I will tell you about a few ideas that I have found productive in the therapy sessions I have conducted. I hope you will improve them in your new production (Lyotard, 1984, p. 4), in a kind of creative outgrowth of what I have presented. If you like these ideas, you might also look at others in some of my recent writings (Shawver, 1996, 1998a,b, 2000, 2001) as well, of course, as in the chapters by other authors in this book.

The three concepts I will highlight here are *tiotoling, generous listening,* and *positional fluidity.* Please think of these names as mere placeholders for concepts that could be variously named and/or conceptualized, and no doubt will be. I imagine affirmative postmodern therapists doing things such as this in therapy instead of giving advice or authoritarian interpretation that would require research proving one therapy paradigm more effective than another.

Tiotoling

In a passage that much impressed me, Lyotard (1979, pp. 71-72) wrote, "For us, a language is first and foremost someone talking. But there are [forms of language] in which the important thing is to listen, in which the rule deals with audition." Some of my friends and I have come to think of this as "tiotoling" (which is an acronym for Talking In Order To Listen that rhymes with "yodeling"). The person who tiotols asks questions or paraphrases, makes associative comments or even contrasting comments, and gives reminders or makes requests, all in order to invite the other to continue rearranging ideas until something seems to work in the situation at hand.

As you can see, tiotoling is not passive listening. It often involves reminding a speaker of what has been said and rearranging what has been said in order to better observe unnoticed connections.

Generous Listening

Generous listening also fosters paralogy. Because our words have multiple meanings, it is often possible to understand a remark in a variety of ways. When this is the case, it seems to promote paralogy if one assumes that the speaker intended the most coherent and reasonable meaning imaginable. Before I give you an example of generous listening, let me provide an example of *critical listening:*

CLIENT: I think I know how to win him back.

THERAPIST: What do you mean you "think you know"? Either you know or you don't know.

Next is a therapist who is listening more generously to this client:

CLIENT: I think I know how to win him back.

THERAPIST: You have an idea but you're uncertain about it?

This generous therapist simply assumed the most coherent interpretation of the client's remarks, but added an association (i.e., "but you're uncertain about it?"). This concept of generous listening seems similar to Davidson's (1984, p. 197) "Principle of Charity." According to Davidson, we listen with the principle of charity when we make the most of what the speakers are saying, giving the speakers the benefit of all doubt and trying to understand their ideas within the meaning of their terms. Anything less seems to frustrate the paralogy. (Although Davidson's concept of the principle of charity seems identical to generous listening, I have relabeled it because "the principle of charity" sounds demeaning to my ear.)

Positional Fluidity

In a modernist dispute each speaker assumes a position and is loyal to a school of thought, often resisting opposing argument. There is no natural shuffling of ideas. In a postmodern conversation, on the other hand, the positions and goals are much more subtle and fluid. Such fluidity allows people to express doubt, yield to different views (McNamee and Gergen, 1999), and also to rearrange the elements of theory by tailoring them to the varying situations. Positional fluidity is the contrast of role rigidity (Harre and van Langenhove, 1999), exemplified by the teacher who is a teacher to everyone, or the flirt who flirts with everyone—even those who feel romantically unappealing. Participants in paralogy tend to abandon role rigidity for increased positional fluidity.

Positional fluidity, seen only in theory, might lead you to wonder if there are goals in a paralogical form of therapy conversation. Indeed there can be goals, but they emerge in the course of the paralogy and, of course, remain available for redefinition. For example, rather than committing to a specific goal of therapy beforehand, such as "losing weight," it might be decided in the course of the paralogy that the degree of weight loss wanted was not desirable or realistic. In paralogy, goals are often revised and improved.

SUMMARY AND CONCLUSION

The past thirty years has been a long, difficult road for psychotherapy outcome research. In retrospect, it almost seems that in those first, heady days therapists were performing therapy on a flying trapeze without the security net of scientific findings to tell them they were doing OK, thinking always that the research would come along and prop up their approaches, saying their preferred therapy styles were the very best. But the Dodo Bird Verdict shattered that hope and primed our field for the production of more than a handful of skeptical postmodern clinicians, people who called themselves "eclectic." There was a period of disappointment, but the crisis passed and something new and hopeful began to emerge, something I have called here the "postmodern hope". (Sometimes I call it "paralogy," and you might call it something else.)

Whatever it is called, it is a new way of talking together, both among colleagues and between therapists and clients. It allows us to do the best we can by pooling our intelligence and learning to cope with our lack of an empirical base for what we do.

Affirmative postmodernism is beginning to blossom in the margins of our field. It is like a new field of flowers taking root in the barren soil of the dream we lost, the dream that we therapists would one day become scientific practitioners. We probably will never be that, in any rigorous sense of the word, but now there is a new model of therapist as paralogical conversationalist, and the need for proving one kind of therapy over another is beginning to fade.

In place of that search for the very best therapy is a new kind of conversation that represents for me the postmodern hope. It is a new dream that is not deflated by the profound wisdom of the Dodo Bird in Alice's Wonderland.

BIBLIOGRAPHY

Andersen, T. (1991). *The Reflecting Team*. New York: W. W. Norton.

Anderson, H. (1997). *Conversation, Language and Possibilities*. New York: Basic Books.

Anderson, H. and Goolishian, H. (1992). The client is the expert: A not-knowing approach to therapy. In S. McNamee and K. J. Gergen (Eds.), *Therapy As Social Construction* (pp. 25-39). Newbury Park, CA: Sage Publications.

Baudrillard, J. (1983). *Stimulations*. New York: Simiotext.

Beutler, L. E. (1991). Have all won and must all have prizes? Revisiting Luborsky et al.'s verdict. *Journal of Consulting and Clinical Psychology* 59(2):226-232.

Carroll, L. (1946). *Alice's Adventures in Wonderland* (Special Edition). New York: Random House.

Chessick, R. D. (1995). Poststructural psychoanalysis or wild analysis? *Journal of the American Academy of Psychoanalysis* 23(1):47-62.

Cushman, P. (1990). Why the self is empty: Toward a historically situated psychology. *American Psychologist* 45(5):599-611.

Cushman, P. and Gilford, P. (1999). From emptiness to multiplicity: The self at the year 2000. *Psychohistory Review* 27(2):15-31.

Davidson, D. (1984). *Inquiries into Truth and Interpretation*. New York: Oxford University Press.

Eysenck, H. J. (1952). The effects of psychotherapy: An evaluation. *Journal of Consulting Psychology* 16:319-324 .

Eysenck, H. J. (1966). *The Effects of Psychotherapy*. New York: International Science Press.

Fiedler, L. (1971). *The Collected Essays of Leslie Fiedler, Volume II*. New York: Stein and Day.

Gergen, K. J. (1990). Toward a postmodern psychology. *Humanistic Psychologist* 18(1):23-34.

Gergen, K. J. (1995). Postmodern psychology: Resonance and reflection. *American Psychologist* 50(5):394.

Gergen, K. J. (1999). *Invitation to Social Construction*. London: Sage Publications.

Glass, J. M. (1993). *Shattered Selves: Multiple Personality in a Postmodern World*. Ithaca, NY: Cornell University Press.

Glover, J. (1926). Divergent tendencies in psychotherapy. *British Journal of Medical Psychology* 6:93-109.

Harms, E. (1970). Historical background of psychotherapy as a new scientific field. *Diseases of the Nervous System* 31(2):116-118.

Harre, R. and van Langenhove, L. (1999). *Positioning Theory*. Malden, MA: Blackwell.

Hassan, I. (1970). Frontiers of criticism: Metaphors of silence. *Virginia Quarterly* 46(1).

Hoffman, L. (2001). *Family Therapy: An Intimate History.* New York: W. W. Norton.

Howard, K. I., Krause, M. S., Saunders, S. M., and Kopta, S. M. (1997). Trials and tribulations in the meta-analysis of treatment differences: Comment on Wampold et al. (1997). *Psychological Bulletin* 122(3):221-225.

Howe, I. (1959). Mass society and post-modern fiction. *Parhsan Review* 26:420-436.

Hynan, M. (1981). On the advantages of assuming that the techniques of psychotherapy are ineffective. *Psychotherapy: Theory, Research and Practice* 18(1): 11-13.

Jensen, J. P., Bergin, A. E., and Greaves, D. W. (1990). The meaning of eclecticism: New survey and analysis of components. *Professional Psychology: Research and Practice* 21:124-130.

Karpman, B. (1947). Psychotherapy. Minor and major. *Quarterly Review of Psychiatry and Neurology* 2:553-577.

Klein, M. H. (1995). Between a boulder and a hard place: The dialectics of positivism, constructivism and hermeneutics. *Humanistic Psychologist* 23(3):305-320.

Lambert, M. E. and Bergin, A. E. (1994). The effectiveness of psychotherapy. In A. E. Bergin and S. L. Garfield (Eds.), *Handbook of Psychotherapy and Behavior Change.* New York: Wiley.

Larsen, D. J. (1999). Eclecticism: Psychological theories as interwoven stories. *International Journal for the Advancement of Counseling*, 21:69-83.

Levin, H. (1960). What was modernism? *Massachusetts Review* 1(4):271-295.

Lionell, M. (2000). Sullivan's anticipation of the postmodern turn in psychoanalysis. *Contemporary Psychoanalysis* 36(3):393-410.

Luborsky, L. (1995). Are common factors across different psychotherapies the main explanation for the Dodo Bird Verdict that "Everyone has won so all shall have prizes"? *Clinical Psychology: Science and Practice* 2(1):106-109.

Luborsky, L., Singer, B., and Luborsky, L. (1975). Comparative studies of psychotherapies. *Archives of General Psychiatry* 32:995-1008.

Lyotard, J. F. (1979). *Just Gaming.* Minneapolis: University of Minnesota Press.

Lyotard, J. F. (1984). *The Postmodern Condition: A Report on Knowledge.* Minneapolis: University of Minnesota Press.

Lyotard, J. F. (1992). *The Postmodern Explained to Children.* London: Turnaround.

Lyotard, J. F. (1993). *Towards the Postmodern.* Atlantic Highlands, NJ: Humanities Press.

Martin, J. (1995). Against scientism in psychological counseling and therapy. *Canadian Journal of Counseling* 29(4):287-307.

Maultsby, M. C. Jr. (1968). Seven reflections on scientism and psychotherapy. *Psychological Reports* 22(3):1311-1312.

McNamee, S. and Gergen, K. (1992). *Therapy As Social Construction.* Newbury Park, CA: Sage Publications.

McNamee, S. and Gergen, K. (1999). *Relational Responsibility: Resources for Sustainable Dialogue.* Thousand Oaks, CA: Sage Publications.

Newman, F. and Holzman, L. (1996). *Unscientific Psychology: A Cultural-Performatory Approach to Understanding Human Life.* Westport, CT: Praeger.

Newman, F. and Holzman, L. (1997). *The End of Knowing: A New Developmental Way of Learning.* London: Routledge.

Ornstein, P. H. (1968). Toward a revised social science: A distinction between two kinds of knowledge. *Psychotherapy: Theory, Research and Practice* 5(1):58-59.

O'Sullivan, J. J. and Quevillon, R. P. (1992). 40 years later: Is the Boulder model still alive? *American Psychologist* 47(1):67-70.

Peterson, D. R. (2000). Scientist-practitioner or scientific practitioner? *American Psychologist* 55(2):252-253.

Phillips, J. (1998). Commentary on "relativism and the social-constructivist." *Philosophy, Psychiatry, and Psychology* 5(1):55-59.

Raimy, V. (Ed.) (1950). *Training in Clinical Psychology.* New York: Prentice-Hall.

Rennie, D. L. (1994). Human science and counseling psychology: Closing the gap between research and practice. *Counseling Psychology Quarterly* 7(3):235-250.

Robinson, D. N. (2000). Paradigms and "the myth of framework": How science progresses. *Theory and Psychology* 10(1):39-47.

Rorty, R. (1979). *Philosophy and the Mirror of Nature.* Princeton, NJ: Princeton University Press.

Rosenau, P. M. (1992). *Postmodernism and the Social Sciences: Insights, Inroads, and Intrusions.* Princeton, NJ: Princeton University Press.

Rosenberg, B. and White, D. (1957). *Mass culture: The popular arts in America.* Glencoe, IL: Free Press.

Schwartz, J. (2000). Further adventures with Adolf Gruenbaum: Response to Gruenbaum. *Psychoanalytic Dialogues* 10(2):343-345.

Seligman, M. E. P. (1995). The effectiveness of psychotherapy: The *Consumer Reports* study. *American Psychologist* 50:965-974. Available World Wide Web: <http://www.apa.org/journals/seligman.html>.

Shadish, W. R. and Sweeney, R. (1991). Mediators and moderators in meta-analysis: There's a reason we don't let dodo birds tell us which psychotherapies should have prizes. *Journal of Consulting and Clinical Psychology* 59(6):883-893.

Shawver, L. (1983). On the disadvantages of assuming that the techniques of psychotherapy are ineffective: A reply to Hynan. *Psychotherapy: Theory, Research and Practice* 20(2):254-256.

Shawver, L. (1996). What postmodernism can do for psychoanalysis: A guide to the postmodern vision. *The American Journal of Psychoanalysis* 56(4):371-394.

Shawver, L. (1998a). On the clinical relevance of selected postmodern ideas: With a focus on Lyotard's concept of "differend." *Journal of the American Academy of Psychoanalysis* 26(4):617-635.

Shawver, L. (1998b). Postmodernizing the unconscious. *The American Journal of Psychoanalysis* 58(4):361-390.

Shawver, L. (2000). Postmodern tools for the clinical impasse. *Journal of the American Academy of Psychoanalysis* 28(4):619-639.

Shawver, L. (2001). If Wittgenstein and Lyotard could talk with Jack and Jill: Towards a postmodern family therapy. *Journal of Family Therapy* 23:232-252.

Shotter, J. (1992). Social constructionism and realism: Adequacy or accuracy? *Theory and Psychology* 2(2):175-182.

Smith, M. B. (1991). *Psychology and the Decline of Positivism: The Case for a Human Science.* Boulder, CO: Westview Press.

Stiles, W. B. (1995). Stories, tacit knowledge, and psychotherapy research. *Psychotherapy Research* 5(2):125-127.

Strenger, C. and Omer, H. (1992). Pluralistic criteria for psychotherapy: An alternative to sectarianism, anarchy, and utopian integration. *American Journal of Psychotherapy* 46(1):111-130.

Thorne, F. C. (1953). Directive psychotherapy: Theory, practice and social implications. *Journal of Clinical Psychology* 9:267-280.

Young, C. and Heller, M. (2000). The scientific "what!" of psychotherapy: Psychotherapy is a craft, not a science! *International Journal of Psychotherapy* 5(2): 113-131.

Walter, J. L. and Peller, J. E. (2000). *Recreating Brief Therapy: Preferences and Possibilities.* New York: W. W. Norton.

Wampold, B. E., Mondin, G. W., Moody, M. Stich, F. Benson, K., and Ahn, H. (1997). A meta-analysis of outcome studies comparing bona fide psychotherapies: Empirically, "all must have prizes." *Psychological Bulletin* 122(3):203-215.

Wittgenstein, L. (1963). *Philosophical Investigations.* (Translated and edited by G. E. M. Anscombe) New York: The Macmillan Company.

SUGGESTED READINGS

Gergen, K. J. (1990). Toward a postmodern psychology. *Humanistic Psychologist* 18(1):23-34.

Hoffman, L. (2001). *Family Therapy: An Intimate History.* New York: W. W. Norton.

Kuhn, T. (1962). *The Structure of Scientific Revolutions.* Chicago, IL: The University of Chicago Press.

Lyotard, J. F. (1984). *The Postmodern Condition: A Report on Knowledge.* Minneapolis: University of Minnesota Press.

Mental health: Does therapy help? (1995). *Consumer Reports* 60 (November): 734-739.

Newman, F. and Holzman, L. (1996). *Unscientific Psychology: A Cultural-Per-formatory Approach to Understanding Human Life.* Westport, CT: Praeger.
Shawver, L. (2001). If Wittgenstein and Lyotard could talk with Jack and Jill: Towards a postmodern family therapy. *Journal of Family Therapy* 23:232-252.
Wampold, B. E., Mondin, G. W., Moody, M., Stich, F., Benson, K., and Ahn, H. (1997). A meta-analysis of outcome studies comparing bona fide psychotherapies: Empirically, "all must have prizes." *Psychological Bulletin* 122(3):203-215.

Chapter 3

Collaboration Within a Pragmatic Tradition: The Psychotherapeutic Legacy of William James

Jon K. Amundson

Jon Amundson presents a collaborative stance in therapy in terms of the pragmatic tradition, here drawing on the psychological legacy of William James. After mapping the latter's seminal distinction between the "tough" and "tender" minded onto the contemporary debate between scientific/empirical and narrative/constructivist approaches in psychology and therapy, Amundson spells out clear practice guidelines for the pragmatic therapist, including pluralism, utility, and helpfulness. In doing so he notes that the kinds of models, theories, or ideas of interest to a pragmatic therapist are those that get the clinical job done! And here, as therapists, we need to realize that therapeutic models are not clinical reality but are meant to fail us.

In this vision of pragmatic therapy, the concern is not to get it right but to struggle with theory and ideas in the day-to-day practice of therapy. It is this pragmatic stance of *knowing-with* that minimizes the violent imposition of theory on others and best expresses a collaborative spirit in psychology and therapy.

The highest ethical life . . . consists at all times in the breaking of rules which have grown too narrow for the actual case . . . and to act so as to bring about the very largest total universe of good which we can see.

William James
The Moral Philosopher

41

INTRODUCTION

There is a Balinese folk saying, "We have no art; we simply do everything the best we can." Though William James was not Balinese, this saying might well apply to his life. Born in 1842 and living into the twentieth century, William James was an educator, a philosopher, a scientist, and a humanist. Raised in a family who counted among their friends Ralph Waldo Emerson (James's godfather) and nurtured their children with an equal emphasis upon culture and intellect (James took a degree in medicine—but not before studying art), by 1873 James was teaching at Harvard and virtually founded the department, if not the discipline, of psychology. Called a genius by many, James himself qualified genius by simply saying it means little more than perceiving things in an unhabitual way. His less than habitual perceptions have loosened our habits and influenced the lives of many. From his actual students (among them Theodore Roosevelt, Gertrude Stein, and W. E. B. Dubois) and those who have admired his ideas (such as Neils Bohr and Daniel Dennett) to his friends/companions (for example Mark Twain) James was considered a creative teacher and a broad, original thinker (Bjork, 1997; Myers, 1997; West, 1989).

Intellectually restless, James wrote not only in the fields of psychology and philosophy (e.g., *The Principles of Psychology, The Varieties of Religious Experience, The Meaning of Truth*) but wandered into racial justice, imperialism, human consciousness and altered states. For a list of essays, excerpts, and reviews, see <http/www.cc.emory.edu/EDUCATION/mp/james.html>. In his intellectual wanderings James has left a legacy that is characterized by openness to mystery and pursuit of practicality in a world of continual change.

IF THERE WAS A JAMESIAN CLINICAL TRADITION . . .

One hundred years ago William James established himself as the first conscientious objector in the essentialist wars of psychology. Although James did not deplore facts, religious sentiment, strong belief, philosophical speculation, or the fruits of scientific investigation, he was cautious in his relationship with any compelling idea. James wrote in a prose that sought less to edify than simply capture his time in mind, to account for the enduring and temporal values that define a given historical era. In this regard his efforts are as relevant today as they were one hundred years ago. In coping with the challenges of imperialism, racism, war, and the hubris of science he faced many of the same challenges we face in our own professional lives. In discussing the ways psychologists might address their objects of study (people and their lives) clinically or otherwise, James differentiated between two modes of thought—what he saw as the "tough" and the "tender" minded (James [1907], 1992, p. 24). By the "tough" minded, James would point to what today we call the research tradition and empirical trend in clinical practice. Within the tough minded we would find those who espouse random clinical trials and speak of effectiveness, efficacy, and empirically based/supported/validated therapy (Amundson and Gill, 2001). Although scientifically skeptical, James's tough-minded therapists would favor facts, including practices perhaps related to assessment and diagnosis (Amundson, 1998).

Conversely, the expansive and even idealistic sentiments of constructivist and narrative traditions would fit well into James's concept of the "tender" minded. Passion, rhetoric, and the hope for justice, as reflected in the highest human values and aspirations, are what characterize the tender. Where the tough minded favor facts, the tender minded champion a softer vision of people and their lives. Between the tough and the tender exists a gulf—a "differend" (Lyotard, 1984)—which not only challenges the integrity of practice but also represents a perennial source of conflict for professional psychology.

Clinical practice struggles to ground itself in ideas that earn their keep. But of what shall these ideas consist? For the researchers and academicians the practices of psychotherapy must be defined. These practices ought to arise from or result in rules that we can follow. Guidelines for therapy arise not from politics, morals, or philosophical speculation but evidence-based consideration. Yet we all seem to know that there is more to the nature of people than one or another empirically supported practice can contain. The political—or the gendered or the moral—is the personal. If we use the illumination of rigor and empiricism to search only where it casts light, what might we miss?

This debate in modern clinical practice between data- or outcome-based treatment and practices related to justice, humanism, and vision from a Jamesian perspective may be beside the point. Neither perspective is presumed ever to be big enough to answer all of the questions, all of the time. I believe James saw the futility of pursuing "final solutions" (Amundson, 1996), whether or not they are empirically or politically correct. In his tradition of conscientious objection—a tradition he called pragmatism—he did not disparage facts or values per se but was more interested in contextual and immediate concerns. It was the interaction between facts and circumstance, between values and necessity, that mattered to James. For example, James could see how an idea—even one as seemingly fundamental as "gravity"—may be subject to reinterpretation in the company of other ideas. Newton's gravity has grown, matured, and rediscovered itself in relation to high-rise construction, space flight, and telecommunications. Although the same in one way, our conception of gravity is also different in particular and evolving context. Bjork (1997), describing James's pragmatism, said it was neither discontinuous bits of truth nor expansive visions of human nature that counted but a world of "context, pattern, connection, potential, and possibility, all shaped relationally" (p. 267).

Therefore James might suggest that therapists and clinicians have less to say about the good, the absolute, or even the necessary, outside of the particular moment, than has been our tendency. Lacan, Skinner, Maslow, or Gergen may tell us what we are about, but that may not be as relevant as we think to the therapy that we do. James—and the neopragmatists—might see theories, models, or therapeutic approaches less as attempts to get it right than as testimony to how many interesting ways we can think of things. In fact, the pursuit of theory or model advocacy would have been abhorrent to James. It is said that he was horrified by the "closet philosopher" (James, cited in Diggins, 1994, p. 139) and "the club sentiment . . . the stifling atmosphere of all official-dom" (Santanya, 1935, cited in West, 1989, p. 57).

Instead of finding the right idea, joining the right club, or using our models and research, our passion and values to find what is right to believe, "conscientious objectors" (C.O.s) might view knowledge less as a foundation to stand upon than as poetry to inspire (Rorty, 1999). There is always more to reality than what we see. Poetry seeks to inspire us to go beyond the apparent and to implement one idea or another to change the way we relate to our surroundings. Poetry, theories, and therapeutics are engaged not in totalizing our environment (i.e., dealing with everything all at once) but in dealing with the issues that arise, one after another, in human affairs. As a result, clinical practice and clinical theory ought not be a competition to see who will be the correct "poet." In fact, a pragmatic clinician might suggest that instead of being spellbound by *one* poet (i.e., beholden to a particular model), it is much more useful to nurture one's capacity to generally and broadly appreciate poetry. C.O.s suffer from an inability to succumb to *either* the assuredness of science or the inspiration of romanticism. Suffering from problems with attention and concentration, pragmatic clinicians read broadly and sample the "verse" available from many fonts of knowledge. For the C.O. the world is a place less of certainty—neither bounded in its wonder by measurement nor affable description—than of mystery and the moment. Clinically each case is its own; knowledge is useful to the extent it serves, and the therapist is inclined toward being a sincere skeptic and an engaged pluralist.

PLURALISM, SKEPTICISM, AND RADICAL EMPIRICISM—WHAT MIGHT THIS MEAN FOR A COLLABORATIVE THERAPY?

If I am lucky, time may make me look smarter than I am. It is time that will weigh the truth of any belief, but especially my belief that we may be at a great turning point in clinical practice. I believe this turning point will have something to do with a shift from scientism, aesthetics, and moral philosophy toward utility and helpfulness. Not that science, deep thought, morality, and ethics will be abandoned. In fact, such important ideas will serve as the basis for and "editors" of the ways/means that psychotherapists will be useful and helpful to others. The change or turning point I am thinking of has to do with no longer mistaking deep thought and inspirational models of therapy with being helpful. It is a change which abandons the belief that one theory, philosophy, or "special" set of data will permit us to finally rank/classify all human circumstance and as a result therapeutically get it right. It is a change that will not abjure pursuit of ideas, be such pursuit driven by science, religion, politics, or philosophy, but it will not seek from ideas any more than poetic inspiration. By "inspiration" we mean sponsorship of utility—ideas which get some work done in the real world of clinical practice. Problems will dictate what they need, not theories. Ideas will be used to solve problems to the extent they seem able to accomplish some work.

This turning point might be about honoring our best ideas and our best data about people and how we might live while just solving the problems patients bring to us simply, politely, and efficiently. I do not believe any change of this sort, or therapy itself, will ever be easy. In fact, to be efficient and respectful in our work will require a lot of resources and a lot of ideas. It will not be enough for us to choose a model and then think for twenty years enraptured by a poem that is "structural" or "systemic," "biological" and "molecular," "narrative" or "empirically validated." Conscientious objectors are required to think more broadly than such luxury would permit. Pragmatic clinical conviction will require discipline, skeptical observation of our most cherished values, *and* the ability to break rules and stretch theory.

To avoid succumbing to ideas, the C.O. will have to look to last things: where it is we (patient[s] and therapist[s]) want to go. Therapy may have to be subject to the patient's approval and judged by standards more rigorous than theoretical purity. Demands may be placed upon therapy which do not come from the book on the shelf or the team behind the mirror. We will perhaps not be allowed to redouble our therapeutic effort when we have forgotten our case-specific aims, never determined our aims in the first place, or had aims ordained in theory or models. Patients and therapists will collaborate to design their own therapy, out from the material of the broader legacy of knowledge we have regarding problems and solutions.

A change of this sort will also require the courage to fail, and when we do, it should be done graciously and skillfully. The fault will not be in our models, theories, or our patients but ourselves. In fact, concern about failure is probably why our theories and schools of thought claim us so readily. Faced with the possibility of imminent failure, models of therapy offer us comfort if not exculpation. We can find reasons why someone did or did not do the right thing. We can be elegant theoretically but useless practically.

In order to more skillfully fail—and succeed even more so—it is important to think usefully. Thinking usefully requires, I believe, a few pragmatic considerations. Most of us have been trained in the spirit of one or another tradition in psychotherapy. Some function in the spirit of Bowen, Minuchin, or Haley, others in the spirit of White. What, however, might therapy be like in spirit of James? How would the atheoretical pragmatist approach to problem solving and the clinical moment look if William James were behind the mirror? To answer this question too well would betray the very spirit of tentativeness that pragmatism entertains. Therefore, I apologize for the inability of my narrative to feed any real theoretical, procedural, or "how to do it" hunger. No therapy manual will be provided. In fact, I fear it is this very hunger which pragmatism seeks to promote. Ideas are presented not to satisfy hunger but to increase appetite. Richard Rorty (1999), a neo-pragmatist and fellow conscientious objector, has said justice is not the end of struggle; justice is struggle. Pragmatic consideration in clinical practice is not about getting it right but the longing and struggling to get it right, case by case, day by day.

EMPIRICALLY INFORMED THERAPY

In connecting ideas to people, in pursuit of change, there are empirical intimations. All therapy is both pragmatic and experimental. Even with the same models, no two therapies are alike, so adjustments and tinkering with even our favorite/preferred "poems" seems inevitable. This tinkering, however, if undertaken methodically and vigorously, might approximate an empirical process.

Although chance and even the random count for much in therapy, chance always favors the prepared. The events in the lives of our patients contribute much to therapy (Hubble, Duncan, and Miller, 1999). The unique things about each patient and his or her special qualities are important; however, preparedness, vision, and vigilance allow us not only to exploit the capacities of our patients but also to judge the degree to which therapy succeeds. Although much of professional psychology has sought either true empirical means or creative narrative means to therapeutic ends, we might abandon either end of such a continuum in our quest to be helpful.

Each case is an experiment, an N of 1, and empiricism—critical process/outcome thinking—might be reflected less in a specified approach (an empirically validated therapy) than in a process (an empirically informed process).

When we think of therapy and James's radical empiricism, I imagine James would want us to consider why therapists and patients might be in a room together in the first place and what they might have to do to call it therapy. As a radical empiricist James would have been interested in what the words or language of the patients meant: what one thing or another might look like, one way or another, in the real world. For we Jamesians, a word means what it shows itself to be. Therefore, a lot of attention in a pragmatic therapy might be directed to understanding why people are there and what the hopes for the therapy might be. In this pragmatic spirit of therapy we owe some allegiance to our behavioral and solution-focused colleagues. Problem definition and the role of therapy in relation to a problem defined may be central to good clinical practice (Stewart, Valentine, and Amundson, 1991). The following thoughts to guide a therapist and the questions that might be posed to patients involve curiosity and tentativeness (Amundson, Stewart, and Valentine, 1993):

- Why is this patient here? And why now? What events have taken place to bring us together? What in general and what in particular has led to his moment? What might he or she expect of me; What might I expect of myself?
- Why is this moment the time to entertain hopes for something different? What does the patient know, feel, think, or hope that might support the pursuit of therapy? How might he or she have to think/feel for it to be time for therapy? What would I have to believe for therapy to take place? Can we foster mutual beliefs of a therapeutic kind?
- In the patient's application for the "job of therapy," what might be on the patient's "resumé" of skills, resources, hidden or subdominant texts, or potentials? How might we get to speak of these "things" that represent the best of him or her? What would he or she need to know in order to feel up to the task of therapy?
- How might the patient and I prove a problem even exists? Why does the patient believe and should I believe there is a problem? What are the ways the problem shows itself in his or her life? What does the patient fear from therapy and what is his or her hope regarding what would be different, in the light of this or that problem?
- If therapy made a difference then what might it look like? Would we even know change was taking place? If therapy got stronger and the problem weaker, how would we know? If the problem

was bigger than the therapy, how might we know we were "failing"? Would therapist, patient, friends of patient, and co-patients all be able to see success or failure, and would the visions all be similar? If different visions of the problem, the therapy or success or failure existed, could the view of success or failure be sufficiently alike to justify therapy?

Before initiating a process which may or many not turn out to be therapy, these rhetorical concerns might fill the room. Nonetheless it is fair to ask how a pragmatically driven therapy might look. How might it be similar or different from collaborative or respectful therapy of any type? What does the struggle to get it right case to case mean in actual practice? To address these questions, it is important to discuss those principles associated with pragmatic habits of thought and offer illustrations. However, to answer such questions too well betrays what pragmatism really ought to be about. James said that pragmatism differs from other intellectual persuasions in that it is a method, a way of thinking or a process—not a "thing" in itself. That it

> stands for no particular results. It has no dogmas, and no doctrines save its method . . . it lies in the midst of our theories like a corridor in a hotel. Innumerable chambers open out of it. In one you may find a man writing an aesthetic volume; in the next someone on his knees praying for faith and strength; in a third a chemist investigating a body's properties. In a fourth a system of idealistic metaphysics is being shown. But they all own the corridor and all must pass through it if they want a practicable way of getting into or out of their respective rooms. (James, 1907 [1992], in Myers, 1997, p. 98)

As mediator, reconciler, or harmonizer, a pragmatic clinical attitude would be no different from any successful, respectful therapy. However, any successful, respectful therapy would probably reflect some, if not all, of the principles associated with pragmatic habits of thought.

PRAGMATIC CLINICAL PRACTICE

A Pragmatic Therapy Always Starts at the End

James ([1907] 1992) has said pragmatism is the attitude of "looking away from first things, principles, categories, supposed necessities; and of looking toward last things, fruits, consequences, facts" (p. 98). Clinically this requires the ability to answer, case by case, the question "How will we know when we are done?"

Tim, age thirteen, had not been attending school enough and as a result his grades had slipped. His parents' concern was greater than Tim's. Nonetheless, in a respectful, neutral conversation it was ascertained that therapy might be over if (1) school performance improved and/or (2) Tim's parents "coached" or "guarded" him less. The parents' therapeutic hope (1) was joined with Tim's hopes (2) and, fortunately, both were achieved.

Defining outcome may be collaborative or driven by the clinician's expertise and experience. Nonetheless, a proposed outcome must enlist and elicit the energy of the parties involved.

A Pragmatic Therapy Is Always Interested in Both Formal and Operational Diagnosis

"Formal" and "operational" (Cummings and Cummings, 2000) represent the difference between the knowledge we have in the discipline of psychology (formal) and the means to bring such knowledge to the matter at hand in useful, accessible, and cooperative ways (operational). With Tim and his family, this binary process involved knowing something about adolescents, parents, family dynamics, and the exceptional and normative aspects of the individuals involved (formal) and the ability to set an agenda that might invite their participation (operational). The pragmatic clinician knows the difference in this regard between "power over" (clinical exercises of control inherent in role and status and formal diagnosis) and "power to" (the ability to efficaciously bring about consequences, operational diagnosis) and favors the latter.

The therapist suggested that the issue for Tim and his family was a regular sort of problem with which most kids had to struggle. This problem was called "drift"—reflected in the adolescent just drifting along rather than steering his or her own life. But not to worry, the therapist "was pretty sure Tim could get normal again."

Although provocative, this "intervention" in fact operationalized what psychology knows about common factors and principles of change.

A Pragmatic Therapy Sees Theory/Models Less As Inherently Effective Than As Vehicles for Common Factors and General Principles Associated with Change

All therapies succeed some of the time, and professional psychology suggests this is because common factors and general principles related to change exist (Hubble, Duncan, and Miller, 1999; Fishman, 1999; Beutler, 2000; Gottman, 1994). Although a diverse literature exists (Amundson and Gill, 2001), good therapy seems to involve

> an emotionally charged confiding relationship between patients and therapists; warmth, support, and attention from the therapist in a "healing" setting; a positive therapeutic alliance between therapist and patient; a new rationale or conceptual scheme offered with confidence by the therapist, "ritual" and the passage of time. (Fishman, 1999, p. 216)

Therefore, rather than enshrine one conceptualization or another concerning theories about the way people work—the way people ought be—and then calibrating therapy accordingly, pragmatic clinicians are always tentative and observant.

Consequently, a Pragmatic Therapy Is Always Experimental and Employs Critical Empirical Process with Each Case

Psychotherapy is to clinical psychology what oncology is to medicine. Treatment of cancer ranges from the highly specified to the experimental but is always governed by the fearsomeness and tentativeness of the disease. In cancer there are cure rates determined by type, onset of disease, time of diagnosis, comorbid conditions, response to treatment, demographics, epidemiology, and morbidity. Psychotherapy ought be similar in its considerations.

Progress with Tim was initially abbreviated and tentative. In our fifth session, in fact, the "therapy" itself was placed center stage. What had happened? In what way? What evidence could the mother, father, or Tim offer to justify more therapy? What counted for evidence? How should we look at what happened, so far, as evidence for or against keeping continuing therapy? While able to justify and account for some progress, the parents were at odds regarding approach. Tim had been diagnosed with ADD but the family felt ambivalence regarding biomedical treatment. The therapist suggested that sometimes medication was at least a partial "antidote to the poison of drift." With such rhetorical framing, the family experimented with its introduction. As result Tim's hopes and his parents' hopes became even more real as his school improved even more.

A pragmatic clinician can neither tell you why you should take medicine nor why you should not. Final or absolute answers cannot be provided except in relation to the reality they serve: Tim went to school and worked harder.

Finally, a Pragmatic Therapy Embraces the Hippocratic Oath of Psychology: "To Neither Deceive nor Be Deceived" by the Methods We Employ

All of us hope for "final solutions" (Amundson, 1996), clinical methods so sure and so true that they will serve our discipline and our patients, always. In our deepest wishes, however, we are vulnerable to believing too much. While we must be passionate, even persuasive, in our efforts, we ought also to be tentative. Psychologists have been wrong before, and we will be wrong again.

Tim and his family went on, apparently better for the consult. Tim and his parents got along better and school improved. A few years later they revisited the therapist. The mother shared how Tim was doing fine. However, "after awhile" he had discontinued his medication, and when, as a family, they reminisced about the therapy, Tim was sure it had not been useful, that he had "just changed." The mother, however, felt that the therapists' work had been useful, in fact that is why they had returned with a young sibling.

Common factors and general principles? Cognitive reframe and behavioral strategies? Ritalin? Good luck? Or good therapy? All that can really be said is that we knew when we were done with Tim and when a new therapy might need to be started for someone else.

CONCLUSION

Outcome, respect, critical attention to process, and collaborative experimentalism characterize a pragmatic therapy. Such a therapy not only realizes that we have enough theories and models but also champions William James's lament of a 100 years ago:

> What can any superficial theorist's judgment be worth, in a world when every one of hundreds of ideals has its special champion already provided in the shape of some genius expressively born to feel, and to fight to the death on its behalf. (James, 1931, pp. 207-208)

Perhaps with the humility of a more pragmatic orientation in our work we can leave theories and models behind, and just be useful.

REFERENCES

Amundson, J. (1996). Why pragmatics is probably enough for now. *Family Process* 35:473-486.

Amundson, J. (1998). Tales of suffering and complaint: Asking DSM-IV to do more than it was intended for. *Journal of Systemic Therapy* 17(3):1-11.

Amundson, J. and Gill, E. (2001). Empirically supported therapies, treatment, guidelines and manual "labor": Hey, wait a minute I just thought of something else! *Psymposium* 10(5):14-18.

Amundson, J., Stewart, K., and Valentine, L. (1993). Temptations of power and certainty. *Journal of Marital and Family Therapy* 19:111-123.

Beutler, L. (2000). David and Goliath: When empirical and clinical standards of practice meet. *American Psychologist* 55:997-1007.

Bjork, D. (1997). *William James: The Center of His Vision.* Washington, DC: American Psychological Association.

Cummings, N. and Cummings, J. (2000). *The Essence of Psychotherapy: Reinventing the Art in the New Era of Data.* San Diego, CA: Academic Press.

Diggins, J. (1994). *The Promise of Pragmatism.* Chicago, IL: University of Chicago Press.

Fishman, D. (1999). *The Case for Pragmatic Psychology.* New York: New York University Press.

Gottman, J.M. (1994). *What Predicts Divorce.* Hillsdale, NJ: Erlbaum Associates.

Hubble, M., Duncan, B., and Miller, S. (1999). *The Heart and Soul of Change: What Works in Psychotherapy.* Washington, DC: American Psychological Association.

James, W. (1891). The moral philosopher and the moral life. *International Journal of Ethics* 1:330-354. Reprinted in Diggins, J.P. (1994). *The Promise of Pragmatism.* Chicago: University of Chicago Press.

James, W. (1931). The Will to Believe and Other Essays in Popular Philosophy. New York: Longman/Green.

James, W. ([1890] 1950). *The Principles of Psychology, Volume I and II.* New York: Dover Publications, Inc.

James, W. (1975). *The Meaning of Truth.* Cambridge, MA: Harvard University Press.

James, W. (1976). *The Varieties of Religious Experience.* New York: Collier Books.

James, W. ([1907] 1992). Pragmatism: A new name for some old ways of thinking. In D. Olin (Ed.), *Pragmatism in Focus* (pp. 13-142). New York: Routledge.

Lyotard, J.F. (1984). *The Post-Modern Condition.* Minneapolis, MN: University of Minnesota Press.

Myers, G. (1997). *William James: His Life and Thought.* New Haven, CT: Yale University Press.

Rorty, R. (1999). *Philosophy and Social Hope.* London, UK: Penguin Books.

Stewart, K., Valentine, L., and Amundson, J. (1991). The battle for definition: The problem with (the problem). *The Journal of Systemic Therapy* 10(2):21-31.

West, C. (1989). *The American Evasion of Philosophy: A Genealogy of Pragmatism.* Madison, WI: University of Wisconsin Press.

SUGGESTED READINGS

Fishman, D. (1999). *The Case for Pragmatic Psychology.* New York: New York University Press.

Gilovich, T. (1991). *How We Know What Isn't So: The Fallibility of Human Reason in Everyday Life.* New York: Free Press.

Hubble, M., Duncan, B., and Miller, S. (1999). *The Heart and Soul of Change: What Works in Therapy.* Washington, DC: American Psychological Association.

James, W. ([1890]1950). *The Principles of Psychology, Volumes I and II.* New York: Dover Publications, Inc.

West, C. (1989). *The American Evasion of Philosophy: A Genealogy of Pragmatism.* Madison, WI: The University of Wisconsin Press.

Chapter 4

Knowing More Than We Can Say

Stephen Frosh

Stephen Frosh's chapter challenges postmodern therapists to re-think the notion that words and language are the sole elements of any therapy. Focusing on systemic family therapy, Frosh celebrates the more conversational and collaborative aspects of the linguistic turn, but asks whether it risks relational violence by ignoring what may be most important to persons in therapy: the unknowable, unsayable, or unsaid. Applying a psychoanalytic lens, Frosh's thesis is that in the process of shedding expertise, technique, and power, postmodern therapists are subject to greater anxiety about what is strange, horri-ble, and demanding in the therapy encounter. In effect, the relinquish-ing of modern structures that defines the postmodern means the un-structured and unnameable in therapy is harder to contain and bear.

The chapter concludes with a fascinating and disturbing evocation of T. S. Eliot's poem "The Waste Land," followed by a dark journey into trauma and Holocaust testimony. This reminds us that therapy con-cerns foremost that of which we cannot speak, which honors the other in an act of knowing that is ultimately an unknowing. In effect, therapy begins where words and knowing fail us and to recognize this is to be collaborative in the truest sense of the word.

Over the course of a number of papers on family therapy and on psychoanalysis (Frosh 1995, 1997, 1999, 2001), I have argued that psychotherapists are mistaken to think that the "postmodern turn" in psychology and psychotherapy means that narrative and dis-course—what can be put into words—are the sole elements of thera-peutic practice. Rather, postmodernism demonstrates the limits of language; how, being encaged within it, its insufficiencies are what we struggle with. Something escapes words, and this "something" is probably what people are most in pursuit of, and most pursued by.

In this chapter, I want to return to this argument and try to think a little more about how a set of relationships concerning what is said, what can be said but is not said, and what is radically unsayable might manifest itself in therapy. I have been led back to this again by another encounter with modernism (Frosh, 2002), which I think has had egregiously bad press among the fashionable exponents of postmodernism, particularly perhaps postmodern psychotherapists. I will come back to this at the end of the chapter, through an example from literary culture, T. S. Eliot's (1922) "The Waste Land"—the most influential poem of the last century—which has again raised for me the futility of any assertion that "language says it all." I will try to examine this through the lens of Ellman's (1990) examination of how the poem intermixes with the insights being developed at the same time by Freud. What becomes key through this examination is a group of issues around language, certainly, but also around silence, memory, fragmentation, abjection—that is, issues which make the unsaid and the unsayable into the most potent, most poignant ghosts at the feast.

POSTMODERN DISCOURSE

First, however, is the main body of my argument, with a particular focus on family systems therapy, which seems to have become the therapeutic enterprise most available to the postmodern and discursive. There is little doubt that postmodernism has revolutionized family systems theory. Gone is the fascination with the machine metaphors that dominated in the early days (cybernetics, systems, homeostasis); lessened is the training emphasis on specific techniques to impact upon the family system—hypothesizing, circular questioning, task setting, paradox. What is "in" now, at least amongst the most self-conscious of postmodern family therapists, is "second-order cybernetics" (e.g., Jones, 1993): that is, an interest in the ways in which therapists impinge upon the system with which they are working, as opposed to simply observing and manipulating it. This carries with it a focus on reflexivity (the feedback loops between therapists and clients, now made transparent) and power relations. It is also linguistic or, in the jargon, "discursive" in formation. As family systems therapy has become more openly reflexive, with more attention paid to the activities of the therapists themselves, so questions of communication and translation have come to the fore. The performativity or effectivity of language has been recognized, and family therapists have come to think of themselves as specialists in storytelling or "narratology." This has had the effect of relativizing the aims of family systems therapy, something always likely to occur given the foundations of much contemporary systems thinking in social constructionism and its forceful opposition toward realist and positivist epistemologies. On the face of it, a highly critical structure of theory and practice has emerged, in which the therapeutic process is interrogated from the perspective of power relations (usually with a Foucaultian gloss); the arbitrariness of any one perspective on experience is stressed so as to allow the emergence of alternative, "subjugated" discourses; the actions of the therapeutic team are democratized and made available to inspection and scrutiny; the creative prospects of language are highlighted; and structural aspects of difference—particularly gender and race—are made central to therapeutic concerns. And although this is not all due to postmodernism, postmodernist thinking is a major influence, particularly because it heightens awareness of the demise of expertise and of grand theory and displaces all truth claims in a manner that seems especially well attuned to the confusions and arguments of psychotherapeutic encounters with couples, families, and other such systems.

It is not part of my concern here to devalue this point of view. In fact, I am very keen on many of these developments in systems theory and think that, along with some parallel developments in psychoanalysis, they have radicalized the possibilities for a critical approach to psychotherapy. The concern of many systems therapists to build their work on the basis of antiracist and antisexist positions, with their concomitant awareness of the ethnocentricity and gender bias present in most Western psychotherapies, seems to me a plausible move forward in a generally progressive direction and well worth supporting. In relation to training as well as therapy it has also been an eye-opener to consider the learning task as one involving the opening out of trainees' perceptions and ways of trusting themselves, rather than incorporating knowledge or learning skills (though I have to say I still demand both of trainees). Certainly my own supervision groups and those of the family systems therapists with whom I have worked have become much more conversational and less directive over the years, more respectful of the positions of the trainees and of the families with whom they are working, and very concerned with the impact of each participant in the therapeutic exchange (family, therapists, team, supervisor) on the other participants. Even if this is not always perfectly achieved, it is more tolerable and stimulating than the ear-bug days, more emancipating and empowering for families and trainees alike, and both lighter and more creative in tone. In this way, the discourse-centered, postmodernism-influenced strategies of teaching and learning adopted by many systems practitioners represents a genuine challenge to the pedagogic strategies used in most professions and indeed, increasingly as class sizes increase, throughout higher education.

But having said this, I am interested here (hopefully, as always) in what is marginalized or occluded by these developments, what they miss. More strongly, while I think there is genuinely much to be learned from postmodernist theory, family systems approaches have in a sense learned the wrong things; or rather, they have learned what they wanted to learn. These have centered on the issue of how, in contrast to psychoanalysis as represented in the standard family systems view (hierarchical, elitist, expert-centered, and— perhaps most damningly of all—*modernist* in outlook), postmodern family therapy is tentative, playful, democratic, and "not-knowing." It achieves this primarily through a social constructionist view of language—that in the process of speech-acting with one another we make meanings, and hence (corollary) these meanings are open to alteration through more speech. The focus is thus on postmodernism's promotion of linguistic playfulness, the way therapy can provide an arena for de- and reconstruction of versions of reality, explored not just abstractly, but through concrete encounters with other people's articulations of their own versions. The *postmodern* gloss on this is taken to be the claim that *all* knowledge is of this contingent, tentative kind, and that claims to the truth are the pathogens in personal and systemic disturbances. From the individual who believes she or he is the source of all good (or bad) in the world, to national groups intent on their rights, truth claims are the cause of problems. Postmodernist therapy, democratic and deconstructionist in its rhetorical freedom, emancipates therapists and clients alike from their ideological belief in reality by articulating alternatives, widening their field of perception, allowing subjugated narratives to be expressed.

TRYING TO FACE THE UNSAYABLE

My complaint about this in many ways attractive presentation of the postmodern alternative to traditional conceptualizations of psychotherapy is that it misses most of the interesting advances produced by postmodernism itself. To my mind, the most radical discovery of postmodernism is not that reality is constituted in language—a fact known to everyone who has absorbed the lessons of modernism and hence not needing anything "post" to prove it. In the specific context of therapy, for example, reality can hardly be derived from anywhere else; even with the various arrangements of bodies spawned by some "new age" practices, most therapy is of the "talking cure" kind, so changes that occur (if any do) can only be theorized as having been produced in one way or another by words. Rather, the important discovery of postmodernism is that it might be impossible to put into words the things which matter, that all the endless talk that constructs the world has the function of *revolving the unnameable,* of taking pot-shots at something which already has moved on. This is why narratives are interchangeable: not because everything is the same, but because language is self-referential, caught in a closed symbolic circuit. As Freud knew, language only hints at what is there; to think otherwise is to make the psychotic error of confusing words with things. Clearly, postmodernism emphasizes the fluidity and productivity of language in making things happen—its account of language is manifestly not representational, but its point is that under postmodern circumstances the dizzyingly kaleidoscopic permutations of linguistic productivity reflect a greater pressure from the *nonlinguistic* arena, from the power of nonrational and irrational forces to break into everyday life. Language is more hectic now, but neither more nor less real than ever it was.

I am arguing here against the idea that narrative can, of itself, constitute therapy and suggesting that postmodernism reveals this by drawing attention to that which cannot be expressed, what Lyotard (1979, p. 81) calls "the unpresentable in presentation itself." Why should it be, then, that family systems therapy seems so insistently intent on learning only part of the lesson of postmodernism, the part which revels in linguistic play but neglects the consequent insight that there is *another site,* something else at work? My suggestion is that this is because, wrapped up in the disavowal of the expert position, modernist claims to truth and the appropriate deconstruction of hierarchy and avoidance of difference in therapy, there is also somewhat of a fear of facing the unknown, irrational, or chaotic demand of the family or other client who is, potentially or literally, *out of control.* Kristeva (1988) portrays this under the emblem of the "stranger"; postmodernism constantly reinvokes this strangeness as something found inside us and reflected, too, outside; what makes the other feared is precisely this haunting, spectral presence of that which cannot be understood and controlled. From the point of view of therapy, what is particularly painful is that clients—individuals, groups, couples, or families as they may be—not only appear with their strangeness, their out-of-controlness, their questions, but that they also demand of the therapist some recognition, some acknowledgment of what they may be. I know for a fact, if such a thing be possible, that I am not the only therapist, or for that matter the only teacher, to sit in a room with clients or students and discover that I am thinking, "What do they want from me?" Actually, I will even hazard the claim that dealing with the issue of *feeling fraudulent* is the principal challenge facing trainees as they learn to become therapists, and it is an issue that stays, or possibly should stay, with them and us for life. When clients say, "help me, cure me, teach me," what on earth do they want? And why, especially, do they want it from me?

My suggestion is that the symptomatic flight of family systems therapists into a specific, narrow rendering of postmodernism is due to a defensive anxiety about the horror of confronting people's neediness, their *demand,* without the protective armor previously given by the claims to expertise, power, and truth generated by the prepostmodern position. That is, as we know from Isabel Menzies-Lyth (1988) among others, "caring" institutions develop their structures at least in part for defensive reasons, to ward off the anxiety of too close an encounter with the disturbing strangeness of the client. Similar processes occur within the wider structures of professional knowledge: the productions of knowledge are manifestations of power, keeping otherness at bay. Postmodernism goes some way toward stripping this bare, showing how these discursive strategies work, how they both express and obscure as they go along, how they are, in the precise psychoanalytic sense, *symptomatic.* Once you know, however, that your therapeutic "techniques" are ways of defending yourself against pain, what are you to do? One observable strategy of avoidance is to pretend that nothing matters, nothing is real; this is not, however, to my mind, a legitimate rendering of postmodernist thought, and anyway it does not work.

INTO THE THERAPIST

There is always a silver lining, of course; otherwise there would not be much point in representing a perspectival position. One interesting feature of the postmodern turn in family therapy has been the reintroduction of the person of the therapist into the scenario. In many ways, this seems anomalous, in that the "person" or "self" is precisely one of the features of symbolization that goes out of the window when postmodernism enters the house. This has become the conventional postmodernist position: that selfhood is fragmentary, identities dissolve, subjecthood is constituted from the outside. All well and good, I say, and I agree with all the material concerning the discursive construction of self and subjectivity; but along with many people—some feminists (e.g., Benjamin, 1998), some social theorists (e.g., Giddens, 1991), some therapists—I want to know what to do to *fill the gap* when my self dissolves in the face of another's demand.

Again thinking symptomatically, I take systemic theory's move back into the arena of the person of the therapist as signifying a wish to manage anxiety. However, here it seems to me there is something not only of a return but also of a next step for postmodernism in its interchange with psychotherapies. In terms of theoretical affiliations, what is happening is that psychoanalysis is coming back onto the agenda. This is rather surprising, given that the first generations of family therapists on the whole repudiated psychoanalysis as precisely the brand of individualistic, privatizing, elitist, and decontextualized practice that they wished to challenge. Thus, despite the efforts of a relatively small number of psychoanalytically inclined family therapists to keep the flag flying, psychoanalytic concerns and psychoanalytic language have been routinely expunged by systemic thinkers. Recognizing this, for example, Anne McFadyen (1997, p. 241) begins an article on the possibilities of "rapprochement" between family therapy and psychoanalysis with the comment that "the relationship between the two disciplines is more often characterized by suspicion than respect." Nevertheless, despite this history, psycho-analysis is making a comeback in many areas of family systems therapy and training. Indeed, McFadyen's paper is one of a series in a special issue of the main British journal for family therapists *(Journal of Family Therapy)* devoted to the topic. There are many aspects of this renewed interest that should excite comment, including the postmodern convergence of both psychoanalysis and family systems theory on questions of language, the place of the inarticulable or "unconscious" in subjectivity, and the question of the relationship between psychoanalytic and systemic concepts of intersubjectivity. However, the one that seems to me most "lived" in practice and most apposite from the point of view of the filling-out of the postmodern vision in psychotherapy, is the question of what goes on "inside" the therapist, or perhaps more precisely what the therapist can draw on in order to respond to the situation to which she or he is subjected (I use the term advisedly). As the postmodern turn displaces issues of technique and structure from the center of therapy (for example, how to ask questions or deliver messages, when to demand that the whole family attend sessions together), so family therapists are being thrown back on themselves and want to know not just what to do, but what it means and how to survive it. What is the "it" here if not the "strangeness" mentioned earlier, the force of the clients' demands, their wish for recognition, their hope for a response?

In a very provocative series of writings, Carmel Flaskas (e.g., 1997; Flaskas and Perlesz, 1996) has reintroduced psychoanalytic ideas such as transference, countertransference, and projective identification into family therapy—and gained a readership by doing so. Without debating her specific use of these notions here, it is worth reminding oneself what they are about. Transference and countertransference, especially as used in British Kleinian theory, refer to the ways in which clients project aspects of themselves into the therapist, eliciting specific emotional and cognitive responses which are then used by the therapist to inform her or his understanding of what is happening. They are thus dynamic ideas referring to the intersubjective exchange that is at the heart of psychotherapy. Projective identification is another mechanism whereby the client stays in touch with parts of her or his self that have become "lost" inside the therapist. What is going on here, then, in this sophisticated return to psychoanalysis bolstered by a thoroughgoing immersion in postmodern tendencies (many of those using psychoanalysis are amongst the most progressive of family therapists), is an attempt to draw into post-modern family therapy a language of, and concern with, interpersonal encounters that can harness the therapist's "self," however fragmentary it may be or become, and enable her or him to respond. In practice, in my own therapeutic work and with my trainees, I keep asking, "how does that feel, what could that feeling mean, from whereabouts in you can you find something to give back?"

To keep this from getting too romanticized, let me review. I have argued that postmodernism has a complex set of messages relevant to psychotherapy, some of which, including its fascination with linguistic productivity and antagonism toward grand truth claims, have been embraced by many therapists. Postmodernism, however, does not stop there but asserts that behind the slippery surfaces of language and image lies an altogether more troubling and fragmenting dimension of experience, with which each of us struggles and which often disturbs and sometimes destroys. This dimension appears in therapy in the form of the subject's "question"; responding to it is a challenge that can be met only through the therapist's willingness to reflect on the internal resonances that it produces. The gap in postmodern family therapy is the relative lack of formal appreciation of this dimension of unspoken trouble; but what it throws back into postmodernism proper is a plea for a theory that is concerned not only with structure and surface but also with the growth of capacities to live with and treat one another just as if we were real.

TOWARD PRACTICE

To conclude, I want to stage a reminder that the concerns with which I have been working—on the margins of language and what can be most powerfully expressed through being left unsaid—are not new, but to a considerable degree dominated the modernist culture of most of the last century, of which postmodernism is just the latest outcropping. In large part, the sense of terror and dissolution around which modernism played, and out of which much of its artistic and psychotherapeutic response arose, was connected with the destructiveness emitted through World War I—a devastating blow to any belief that scientific rationality was leading the West forward to a more civilized future. The supposed dominance of reason was in fragments and the power of irrationality, of what had previously been thought (and through Freud continued to be thought) as "primitive" unreason, had been clearly demonstrated. In Britain, by the mid-1920s, the nature of the war was very well known and its consequences had been felt across an entire generation. Everything had changed and had to change. T. S. Eliot's "The Waste Land" (1922), despite or perhaps alongside its misogyny and reactionary class bias, grabbed hold of this feeling and represented it with appalling precision, in a manner congruent with the emerging discipline of psychoanalysis. Ellman (1990), in a marvelous examination of the poem's "abjection" (a concept taken from Kristeva, 1983), comments on wiping out a history which then returns, plaguing the text, like the return of the repressed which in Freud is the prototype of death: "Whereas Freud discovers the death drive in the compulsion to repeat, *The Waste Land* stages it in the compulsion to citation" (Ellman, 1990, p. 188).

> *The Waste Land* works like an obsessive ceremonial, because it re-inscribes the horrors it is trying to repress. For Freud argues that obsessive rituals repeat the very acts that they are thought to neutralize: the ritual, he says, is ostensibly a protection against the prohibited act; "but *actually* . . . a repetition of it." (pp. 179-180)

The "waste" in "The Waste Land" is what constantly returns, the living dead; the ghosts and fragments, of people and particularly of writing.

> [T]he abjection of *The Waste Land* arises out of the displacements which haunt it from within: the mutual contamination of the past and present, of the dead letter and the living voice. Eliot's quotations demonstrate how written signs are necessarily displaceable, orphaned from their origins and meanings . . . Beneath the meaningful connections of the text a parodic underlanguage opens forth, based on the contagion between sounds. (pp. 192-193)

Here we have both the exquisite pain of linguistic, discursive representation and the calling into being of an underside, what Ellman calls an "underlanguage," that subverts and displaces it. "The Waste

Land" is a particularly powerful instance of a widespread modernist dismay at the failure of reason and memory to hold in check the ghosts of irrationality; its fragmentary nature and plague of citations ("the rattle of its own exhausted idioms" [Ellman, 1990, p. 192]) perform the boundaries of its own linguistic expressiveness, evoking what cannot be said yet is all too irrevocably there. Similarly, I suggest, with psychotherapy: where words fail is often where therapy begins. Obviously, much of the work entails wresting into language that which usually is unspoken, whether through bad faith or trauma; but a point to recall is that in and amongst all the linguistic interchange, all the discursive reproduction, when people sit together to talk about important things, they are haunted by ghosts, "like the spirits flowing over London Bridge, the restless corpses and the hooded hordes" (Ellman, 1990, p. 197). These are things unspoken and sometimes unspeakable, with which we do our best.

Thinking about how this might relate to the actual practice of relational nonviolence in therapy, I want to focus briefly on the avoidance of a coercive "knowing" as we are faced with the impact of distress. The paradigmatic case here is that of trauma, in which the failure fully to symbolize experience is a main part of the definition, and which has now, arising out of psychoanalytic studies of Holocaust testimony (Felman and Laub, 1992), spawned a whole area of study—trauma studies. As Bennett and Kennedy (2003) note, this work has "drawn our attention to the need to seek out testimony, to recognize its expression in non-narrative languages that convey the affective nature of trauma, and to read the gaps and silences which necessarily accompany the process of testifying" (p. 3). Sometimes this is a "therapeutic" move, but at other times putting the trauma into words can disrupt a hard-won stability that *depends on* silence: "The representation of memory is not always restorative—far from it, especially when it concerns the integrity of the body. Memory may suddenly destabilize, and words may prove to be the site of that undoing" (Scott, 2003, pp. 83-84). I have made a similar point previously (Frosh, 2001) in relation to Holocaust testimony, arguing that although it may help many to be given the opportunity to speak about their experiences, the rationale for testimony gathering is not, in the end, a therapeutic one. The example I used comes from Claude Lanzmann's *Shoah,* where, in one of the most evocative sections of the film, the barber Abraham Bomba is describing—or, rather, *reenacting*—his experiences in the gas chamber, something he seems not to have spoken fully of before and cannot bear to do now. As the story is drawn out of him by Lanzmann ("You have to do it. I know it's very hard. I know and I apologize") it becomes clear that the articulation of the experience is not being done for the sake of the testifier or witness, but in order to bring something to life for the *listener,* who has to know it. From the witness's point of view, preserving a nondiscursive space for his experience has been a simple and significant act of survival.

What dictates the difference here between trauma eased by speech and trauma maximized by it is probably a mixture of the power of the experience itself and of the context in which the witnessing takes place. Apfelbaum (2001) argues compellingly that what matters is both the social context making speech possible (in the immediate aftermath of World War II, the concentration camps *could not* be spoken of) and the capacity of a listener to hear ("It takes two to speak the truth," p. 28). Apfelbaum describes the range of strategies brought into play by listeners who avoid facing the story of trauma and its impact, and stresses the leap of imagination required to keep to the open, "not knowing" stance that might lie at the basis of all truly restorative therapy.

> The only way to truly hear a survivor's narrative is by entering the alien world of the narration. It is, therefore, to abandon one's safe framework and no longer pretend to know/understand within that framework. But it is also to acknowledge the essential difference between the speaker's world and that of the listener . . . The only way to truly hear is to acknowledge the unbridgeable gap between the two worlds, and to assimilate the impact of this unbridgeable difference. Understanding is irrelevant (the reality always exceeds what the narrative is able to represent and convey). What is important is the willingness to become part of the transmission. (p. 30)

With our trainees and with ourselves, what offers hope for a move forward into a practice that recognizes the existence of this otherness is a constant reiteration of the message that we can know more than is said, even if we can only know it through hints and possibilities. Part of this act of knowing requires a deep reflection on the impact of the client's story upon us—hence the relevance of the reflexive position and the concepts taken from psychoanalysis. Another part of it relates to constant scrutiny of the honesty of our response. A further, and perhaps the most important and difficult part, is connected with a stance of not trying too hard; that is, not hoping to understand everything or believing that one can, but nevertheless, in the heart of that not-understanding, reflecting back to the other both her or his difference and the willingness that the therapist might have to stay in this impossible dialogue.

REFERENCES

Apfelbaum, E. (2001). The Dread: An Essay on Communication Across Cultural Boundaries. *International Journal of Critical Psychology 4:*19-34.

Benjamin, J. (1998). *Shadow of the Other: Intersubjectivity and Gender in Psychoanalysis.* New York: Routledge.

Bennett, J. and Kennedy, R. (2003). Introduction. In J. Bennett and R. Kennedy (Eds.), *World Memory.* London: Palgrave.

Eliot, T.S. (1922). "The Waste Land." In *The Waste Land and Other Poems* (pp. 61-86). London: Faber, 1940.

Ellman, M. (1990). Eliot's Abjection. In J. Fletcher and A. Benjamin (Eds.), *Abjection, Melancholia and Love: The Work of Julia Kristeva* (pp. 179-199). London: Routledge.

Felman, S. and Laub, D. (1992). *Testimony.* New York: Routledge.

Flaskas, C. (1997). Engagement and the Therapeutic Relationship in Family Therapy. *Journal of Family Therapy 19:*263-282.

Flaskas, C. and Perlesz, A. (1996). *The Therapeutic Relationship in Systemic Therapy.* London: Katnac.

Frosh, S. (1995). Postmodernism versus Psychotherapy. *Journal of Family Therapy 17:*175-190.

Frosh, S. (1997). Postmodern Narratives. In R. Papadopoulos and J. Byng Hall (Eds.), *Multiple Voices: Narrative in Systemic Family Therapy* (pp. 86-102). London: Duckworths.

Frosh, S. (1999). What Is Outside Discourse? *Psychoanalytic Studies 1:*381-390.

Frosh, S. (2001). Things That Can't Be Said: Psychoanalysis and the Limits of Language. *International Journal of Critical Psychology 1:*39-57.

Frosh, S. (2002). Psychoanalysis in Britain. In D. Bradshaw (Ed.), *Modernism* (pp. 116-137). Oxford: Blackwell.

Giddens, A. (1991). *Modernity and Self-Identity.* Cambridge, UK: Polity.

Jones, E. (1993). *Family Systems Therapy: Developments in the Milan-Systemic Therapies.* Chichester: Wiley.

Kristeva, J. (1983). Freud and Love. In T. Moi (Ed.). *The Kristeva Reader* (pp. 238-271). Oxford: Blackwell, 1986.

Kristeva, J. (1988). *Strangers to Ourselves.* London: Harvester Wheatsheaf, 1991.

Lanzmann, C. (1985). *Shoah: The Complete Text.* New York: Pantheon Books.

Lyotard, J.F. (1979). *The Postmodern Condition.* Manchester: Manchester University Press, 1984.

McFadyen, A. (1997). Rapprochement in Sight? Postmodern Family Therapy and Psychoanalysis. *Journal of Family Therapy 19:*241-262.

Menzies-Lyth, I. (1988). *Containing Anxieties in Institutions.* London: Free Association Books.

Scott, A. (2003). Language As a Skin. In J. Bennett and R. Kennedy (Eds.), *World Memory.* London: Palgrave.

SUGGESTED READINGS

Frosh, S. (2002). *After Words.* London: Palgrave.

Papadopoulos, R. and Byng Hall, J. (Eds.) (1997). *Multiple Voices: Narrative in Systemic Family Therapy.* London: Duckworths.

Chapter 5

On the Way to "Presence": Methods of a "Social Poetics"

Arlene Katz
John Shotter

Although it is arguable that "theory," in the form of cultural ideas and beliefs, always informs our interactions with one another, it is probably fair to say that this is more the case in the professional domain than it is in our informal relationships. We typically approach our clients, students, supervisors, and research participants "through" theories that help make sense of what we are up to. In doing so, we orient toward others in what might be called an instrumental fashion—that is, we do something *to* them rather than *with* them. Arlene Katz and John Shotter have written extensively about an alternate approach to relating which they have called, among other things, mutual responsiveness, or joint action. Drawing on the work of Ludwig Wittgenstein, Mikhail Bakhtin, and others, they articulate an orientation to practice that, as they say, is less about "having a point of view" and more about responding, utterance by utterance, to that which is given.

We certainly do not mean to suggest that this approach is not theoretically informed—on the contrary, Katz and Shotter are among the most sophisticated and subtle theoreticians writing about counseling and therapy today, as this sometimes challenging chapter will illustrate. But they advocate for a view of therapy that is more akin to conversation than technique, and for practice that is more about responding to the particularities of what clients say than "using a theoretical model." In this chapter the authors draw on a case vignette to provide a rudimentary outline of the methods of what they call a "social poetics."

There are as many different worlds of the event as there are individual centers of answerability. If the "face" of the event is determined from the unique place of a participative self, then there are as many different "faces" as there are different unique places.

Bakhtin, 1993, p. 45

(meaning is a physiognomy)

Wittgenstein, 1953, no. 568

. . . the units of inner speech . . . resemble the alternating lines of a dialogue.

Voloshinov, 1986, p. 38

We begin at the end, with the final reflections of a patient in a primary care family practice, a man in his mid-fifties (Mr. C), on the special nature of the care he had received there. It had involved him in a three-way meeting, both with his primary care physician and with one of us (AK). He had found the whole process of meeting as a team quite unique.[1]

MR. C: I think that [the three-way meeting] was a big difference because now you got two, you know, listening to each other when the three of us are talking. And you know, if one doesn't pick up, I'm sure the other one will.

He remarked that they both had asked different questions, and that that had not only opened up new ideas to think about but also, he felt, given him a new way to answer his questions—"Gee, it's something to think about . . . which I never thought before, you know. I say, '*that's* an idea,' you know . . . yeah, how *did* it come about?" And these questions "traveled." He "carried" them around with him. They kept on opening up new possibilities in his everyday life.

MR. C: A lot of things worked for me. I think in a sense where—even the way you two put it together, you know. It was like, it was like, you know, I had no pressure on. It was like a nice way to go about the situation, you know, from day one. It was very comfortable. And I think that's the key, you know, you have to be comfortable with your doctor . . . I thought it made a difference. And I thought it was unique—which most of my friends, most of the family, they think it's unique, and they think it's different; they think it's nice.

Initially, the man had come to see his doctor, worried that he was unable to go in to work anymore. He had gone from working three jobs and a sixty-hour week to feeling, he said, "extremely nervous . . . I don't sleep anymore . . . I feel in a fog."

What was special about Mr. C's speech, as he talked of his worries and anxieties with either AK or his doctor, was its multivoiced, dialogical structure. He spoke of what his wife, his boss, his father, or even his body, said to him about his worries: "It's like you can only stay still so much—like you are paralyzed. You say to your body, 'Even if you don't want to put pressure on yourself, take a step at a time—you have to do it. You have to go to work. You're getting it out of your system.' Many times my wife says, 'You put barriers out.' I was in a fog; at least I see the world more clearly. I feel like a progression . . ." Reflecting later on how he now feels, he says, "It's like it's two different worlds, doctor. It's like you're in a dark hole, and you're back again in an open world. Big difference, yeah."

MUTUAL RESPONSIVITY

How should we make sense of such an account as this? How might we describe its features in such a way that, in our responses to it, we might learn a "way of looking" which can "travel," in other words, which we can "carry over" into our involvements with other people and clients; responses that will—just as with our questions to Mr. C, which kept on opening up new possibilities for him in his everyday life—open up new possibilities for those of us working as therapists?

There are two possibilities: (1) seeking a theoretical hypothesis, a conceptual framework to explain what happened in the case of Mr. C, in the hope that it will help us make useful interventions, and then to carry over that framework in thinking about other such cases; (2) another, very different approach is suggested by two remarks of Wittgenstein's: the first has to do with us "wrongly expecting an explanation, whereas the solution of [a] difficulty is a description if we give it the right place in our considerations. If we dwell *upon* it, and do not try to get beyond it" (1981, no. 314, emphasis added). The second remark suggests that not just any old description will do; one of a special poetic kind is required. We need a description that "arrests" us, that functions to put a flow of activity on "freeze frame," so to speak, and which then moves us to search it over for ways in which to relate ourselves responsively to aspects of it that we might not otherwise have noticed. What is needed, says Wittgenstein (1953), is "a perspicuous representation {Ger: übersichtlichte Darstellung}," [an expression] "that produces just that understanding which consists in 'seeing connections'" (no. 122). Rather than thinking "about" how to plan an intervention into our circumstances, such poetic descriptions can aid us in becoming more alert, sensitive, and, above all, continuously responsive to connections and relations between events, from within our ongoing involvements.

It is this second possibility that we want to explore in this article. For it is only in how we reveal the "contours" of our ways of being to one another, in the continuous interplay of mutual responsiveness between us, that we become present as the people we are to one another. Consider a handshake: although both involved synchronize their rhythmic movements to an extent, each is responsive to the other in his or her own distinctive way. As a result, in the unfolding "shape" of the subtle variations, between the outgoing rhythmic movements toward the other and the resultant incoming movements, each is *present* to the other in some minimal way.

We are interested, then, not in a stance toward our surroundings, in which a theory is tested in a sequence of discrete, punctuated experiments, but in what occurs when we take a conversational stance which allows us, so to speak, to remain continually "in touch" with our dialogue partner, with the "contours" of his or her being.[2] It is our focus on people's spontaneous responsiveness to the others and othernesses around them that is, we feel, the key feature in our approach.

This process of people becoming present to one another in their interactions is quite familiar to us in our daily lives, but it is unfamiliar to us in social theory. Thus, before we can turn to its exploration, we must first make a number of preliminary points.

We must first note that in considering these two possibilities, the urge to withdraw and to seek explanatory hypotheses in such circumstances is very strong. Given our disciplinary training, it is very easy for us to treat a disorientation or a disquiet as a technical problem, a cause-and-effect problem requiring an intellectually thought-out so-lution. Hence we seek, individually and monologically, to make ex-ternal "interventions." How different it is to offer, dialogically, a partic-ular response to another's actions which might lead to his or her noticing of previously unnoticed connections and relations to his or her present surroundings, and thus to the creation (construction) of new possible ways in which to respond. Thinking of ourselves as wholly self-contained, contemplative individuals (Sampson, 1993) who must deliberate before we act, we do not think of language (speech) as being useful in this attention-directing way. We think of language as having the sole function of transmitting information across the dis-tance separating us from one another. In this theory-seeking stance, we try to influence others through the algorithms, theories, or general in-formational guidelines upon which *we* feel that *they* should base their actions.

This, however, is to think of the others around us simply as other things in the world, and to ignore the fact that they are here with us and we are here with them, that we are always in fact to an extent present to one another in an ineradicable, two-way, living relation to one another. Even when attempting to adopt a one-way, interventive relation toward them we rely on this two-way relation continuing in the background if we expect them to understand our questions and to follow our instructions. To think we are in only a mechanical cause-and-effect relation to events in our surroundings is to ignore the cru-cial role of our spontaneous, living bodily responsiveness to the oth-ers and othernesses around us. Indeed, such an intellectual stance stands in the way of us acknowledging the importance of many other features of our mutual spontaneous responsiveness.

Most crucially, it leads us to ignore the first-time creative or consti-tutive function of our expressions. In spontaneously responding to events in our surroundings in a particular and unique way, we also create between ourselves and our surroundings a relationship of a unique and particular kind—and it is from within such unique rela-tionships, once established and attuned to the details of a client's life, that everything of therapeutic importance to us occurs. Indeed, we can go further with this "insider," relationally responsive view of things. For we can call those kinds of change in which a person's self as such essentially remains unchanged and in which he or she merely acquires some new knowledge about the world's externally imposed or outer changes, while those changes in which persons are changed in themselves, in their very way of being in the world, we can call internally responsive or inner changes. It is only changes of the second kind, internal changes, originating from within the spaces between us, that are of interest to us here.

FROM FIXITY TO FLUIDITY,
FROM ENTANGLEMENTS TO SELF-RESPECT:
CONVERSATIONAL ETHICS

To the extent that such inner or internally responsive changes are felt as advantageous, we find that they are formulated variously (to paraphrase Mr. C's words) as a movement from dark to light, as a shift from absence to presence, from fog to clarity, from stuckness or fixity to fluidity. Such an enriched practical understanding of the possible connections between events does not necessarily provide us with any new theories for thinking "about" them, but enables us to be more "at home" within our own activities, to know our "way about" (no. 123) within them, and thus to avoid, as both professionals and ordinary folk, becoming "as it were, entangled in our own rules" (no. 125), in other words, to avoid being at cross-purposes with one another, or ourselves.[3] For it is when we are in disagreement with ourselves, so to speak, that we lose our self-respect.

Crucial to our approach, then, is the importance of people relating to one another (and to themselves) in a fully spontaneously responsive fashion. In short, in an intimate way. And as Bakhtin (1986) notes, in such intimate forms of speech, speakers perceive their addressees as "more or less outside the framework of the social hierarchy and social conventions, without rank, as it were. . . . Intimate speech is imbued with a deep confidence in the addressee, in his sympathy, in the sensitivity and goodwill of his responsive understanding. In this atmosphere of profound trust, the speaker reveals his inner depths" (p. 97). Only if people meet one another in this fully mutually responsive fashion, can they have a sense of one another's inner being—the unique individuals they are. And only if people are present to one another in this sense can they affect one another through their interactions in ways that matter. If we are to "make a difference that makes a difference" (Bateson, 1979, p. 78) internally, in the being of those to whom we address ourselves, our expressions or utterances must only be voiced in response to the utterances or expressions of those we address.

When people act in this mutually responsive fashion, with each person's actions partially "shaped" by the other's responsive reactions, something very special happens: they find themselves in an essentially ethically demanding situation. As Bakhtin (1986) points out,

> Each dialogue takes place as if against a background of the responsive understanding of an invisibly present third party who stands above all the participants in the dialogue (partners). . . . The aforementioned third party is not any mystical or metaphysical being (although, given a certain understanding of the world, he can be expressed as such)—he is a constitutive aspect of the whole utterance, who, under deeper analysis, can be revealed in it. (pp. 126-127)

and who functions as "the witness and the judge" (p. 137) of what we say and do within it. At each moment, it is as if the dialogue or conversation itself, as a kind of agent in its own right, decrees the options available to, and limitations upon, those participating in it.[4] We ethically violate the being of our dialogue partners if, in inviting a response by addressing them with a question, we then use their response only in the confirmation or rejection of our own already-adopted, theoretical hypothesis, and are not ourselves responsive to them as they have been responsive to us.

To ignore the conversation's continuously changing requirements, moment by moment, and to insert into it from the outside theoretical requirements of our own, is to claim a legitimacy (a rank, an authority) for ourselves that we deny to them.

ORIENTING IMAGES AND EXAMPLES: METHODS OF A SOCIAL POETICS

We live our lives, then, unavoidably situated within a vast, usually unnoticed, flow of spontaneous living bodily responsiveness to the activities of the others and othernesses around us. Although we do point out and verbally formulate the character of certain selected aspects of this flow of responsive activity, its extensive nature is such that much of it still remains unnoticed and unarticulated in the background to our self-conscious actions.[5] In what follows in this section, we will set out what we see as some of the central methods of what we have called a social poetics, a set of practices "inter-animated" by, or "in-formed" by remarks drawn from Wittgenstein's writings.[6]

We can see these methods at work in what follows. When Mr. C remembered being able to return to work he was struck that, "It was like being back to myself. It was like I never left." In further elaboration he stated, "It gave me energy and dignity that I always had." In dwelling on the word *dignity,* we could now "follow him" as he looked back in order to move forward.

AK: I was struck by your word "dignity" and that it is important to have that back.

MR. C: Ah, very important. I'd watch my neighbors every morning— they'd go to work in their suits and come home—and here I am doing nothing. It brought me down.

Articulating what is at stake for him made visible values that otherwise could have gone unnoticed: "I feel like a man without a country without work. I'm just existing. I got in touch with how much I missed the good things."

A central method here, is noticing the striking moments.[7] This, however, is easier said than done,[8] but a readiness to be "struck" in this way is a part of the "conversational-poetic stance" we shall describe in a moment. By dwelling on such moments we notice new connections, for example, images or metaphors that can become "objects of comparison which are meant to throw light on the facts of our language by way not only of similarities but dissimilarities" (Wittgenstein, 1953, no. 130). Rather than images representing a situation already clear and familiar to us (with which others might or might not agree), these are images "through" which or "in terms" of which we might, for the first time, make a certain kind of sense of previously unnoticed events occurring in our surroundings, a sense that can be shared with others—and later as examplars that can be carried over into other circumstances. Here, Mr. C shifts how he is situated, in time and place—from fixity to movement, dark to light. In doing so he begins to navigate from within what he now feels to be a very different landscape of possibilities.

Let us explore further the poetics of this most important notion of a landscape of possibilities. Metaphorically, two images might seem (on the face of it) to be appropriate in trying to capture the nature of people's situatedness. We might first talk in terms having a place or position in a historically changing time-space (a "chronotope," in Bakhtin's [1981] terms), a position on a landscape, a surface which to an extent could be "looked over" or "surveyed." But we can also talk of being "rooted," not so much in a particular region in space as in a relationally engaged activity. Here, in this more vertically oriented image, the more visible aspects of our activities, on the surface, need to be understood in terms of their less visible "underground" aspects—from which, historically, they have "grown" or developed. Both these images are of importance to us here. Speaking responsively, from within a rooting or a position in the spontaneous flow of shared activities among us all, is clearly quite different from speech divorced from any involvement in such a flow.

In this connection, there is a further image of importance to us: that of the "face" (Bakhtin) or the "physiognomy" (Wittgenstein) of a situation. Our immediate response to facial expressions is very basic. When very young, before any awareness or consciousness of meaning occurs, we spontaneously respond to the facial expressions of those around us in characteristic ways. Indeed, we often use it to capture the way in which we are initially "struck" by a situation: "On the face of it, it seems. . . ," we say—just as we did in our comment in parentheses in the previous paragraph.

Indeed, as Bakhtin (1993) puts it:

> [A]ctual Being-as-event is determined in its uniquely important, heavy, and compellent event sense . . . precisely in correlation with my own obligative uniqueness: the compellently actual "face" of the event is determined for me myself from my own unique place. But if this is so, then it follows that there are as many different worlds of the event as there are individual centers of answerability . . . [and] there are as many different "faces" as there are unique places. (p. 45)

In other words, each moment in a conversation has a "face" or a "physiognomy" that elicits a response from us. It exerts a "compellent" call upon us, an acknowledgment from us as to what is at stake. Thus when Mr. C says that a shift has taken place within him, from being "in a dark tunnel" to being "back again in an open world," it is, we would like to say, the compellently actual "face" of his circumstances that has changed. He can now face his circumstances differently; his "responsive understanding" (Bakhtin, 1986) of them has changed; he is now "situated" quite differently. We are similarly asked to account differently; we are now answerable to him in a different way, and must now acknowledge what is at stake for him differently too.

CONCLUSION:
THE CONVERSATIONAL-POETIC STANCE

Previously, then, in discussing the case of Mr. C, we gestured toward a number of the methods of a social poetics.[9] But these methods cannot be used unresponsively, as if following a checklist. They can be used only in response to our sense of another's presence to us in our interactions with him or her, and they will only have their effect if we are present to them. To hold ourselves open to being responsive to the otherness of the other in a way that allows the possibility of a coming to presence, a special stance or attitude is required—if either stance or attitude is the right word for something so dynamic and complex. We shall call it simply a "conversational-poetic stance." We cannot describe the complex nature of such a stance in much detail here, but suffice it to say that, in contrast to our usual forms of talk, in terms of having a "point of view" and of viewing things in terms of a certain "perspective," such a stance requires each of us to responsively follow the movements of the other wherever they might lead.

In other words, there is a kind of fluidity in conversation that is lacking in a theory-driven inquiry or a debate about ideas. If we are to let "something" speak to us of itself, of its own inner "shape," we need to follow where it leads, to allow ourselves to be moved in a way answerable to its calls. This is what we meant when we suggested that, if we wish another's inner nature to become present to us, instead of dwelling on his or her behavior, we should dwell with him or her. Instead of "investigating" the client according to our own, pre-established theoretical requirements, we must let his or her inner nature reveal itself to us in our caring for and coping with him or her in our lives.

This led us on to a final image that had to do with Mr. C's changed relationships (through a different kind of inner dialogue) to his circumstances. Katz (1991) reports an exchange with a man, D, and his wife, K, following a reflecting team's comments on the relations between them: AK says to D: "So it wasn't only generative in terms of other ideas, it was generative of ideas leading to action." D replies: "Yes. I've used both of those two approaches in the intervening time . . . *I'm aware of being able to do that now.* What it gave me was a kind of new vocabulary or *language to talk to* myself, to say 'wait a minute,' or 'what about . . .?' Or, 'it doesn't have to be perfect, let's take a look at what isn't perfect . . .'" (p. 119). K adds: "Yes. For me it was the delicacy and the close attention and caring" (p. 119). It was the tone, the "music" in their voices, that moved her.

As Voloshinov (1986) comments about our inner speech: "they resemble the alternating lines of a dialogue. There was good reason why thinkers in ancient times should have conceived inner speech as inner dialogue" (p. 38). For as each line of dialogue ends, the next utterance in the dialogue—if it is truly a dialogue—must be in response to the "impression" that line has made on listeners to it, and the two together are thus inevitably creative of a new momentary relationship. Indeed, Voloshinov continues his comments along just these lines:

> These units of inner speech, these total impressions of utterances, are joined with one another and alternate with one another not according to laws of grammar or logic but according to the laws of evaluative (emotive) correspondence, dialogical deployment, etc., in close dependence on the historical conditions of the social situation and the whole pragmatic run of life. (p. 38)

And as with D and K reflecting on the usefulness of hearing a reflecting team's utterances, so Mr. C also found his conversations with his doctor and AK useful in the same way: the "face" of his conversations changed. They did not just give him new ideas, but came to exert quite different "compellent" calls upon him as he "carried" them over into his daily affairs.

We previously wrote that the kind of understanding we were aiming at by the use of these poetic methods did not have to do with arriving at any new theories but was a kind of practical understanding that enabled us to be more "at home" inside our own social creations, to know our "way about" (no. 123) within them, thus to avoid being at cross-purposes—both with the others we meet and with ourselves.

Their aim is not to discover anything new or previously unheard of, but to aim at a kind of clarity in which what had seemed to be a problem "should completely disappear" (no. 133). But this, to repeat, can be achieved only by people being truly dialogically responsive to one another. As soon as one dialogical partner imposes a theoretical scheme on another, and insists that such scheme makes better sense of his or her activities than he or she can, then we are in danger not only of becoming alienated from them but also of becoming alienated from ourselves. It is in the character of our own inner dialogues that we can become both present to others and to ourselves.

NOTES

1. AK was involved in an ethnographic project at the time, to chart the special overall operations of the collaborative nature of the primary care family practice in question, as part of a larger project looking at the changing face of health care. Personal details of the patient have been altered or omitted to preserve confidentiality.

2. The point-by-point testing of theories results in a knowledge framework that as Quine (1953) puts it, "is a man-made fabric which impinges on experience only along the edges" (p. 42). The possibility of people being "present" to one another, in all their unique, "contradictory" complexities, is eliminated in this discontinuous, out-of-touch approach to the acquisition of knowledge.

3. All (no.) only citations are from Wittgenstein (1953).

4. "There are many occasions when the individual participant in a conversation finds that he and the others are locked together by involvement obligations with respect to it. . . . Due to the ceremonial order in which his actions are embedded, he may find that any alternate allocation of involvement on his part will be taken as a discourtesy and cast an uncalled-for reflection upon the others, the setting, or himself. And he will find that his offense has been committed in the very presence of those who are offended by it" (Goffman, 1967, p.115).

5. "Perhaps what is inexpressible (what I find mysterious and am not able to express) is the background against which whatever I could express has its meaning" (Wittgenstein, 1980, p. 16).

6. A complex point is at issue here, one that we cannot properly tackle in the brief compass of this chapter. But by suggesting that the practices in question are "interanimated" or "in-formed" by aspects of Wittgenstein's writings, we wish to draw attention to the special role played by his remarks. A process quite different from the "application" of rules, dicta, or maxims is at issue. At crucial points or moments within our ongoing relations to our surroundings, his remarks work, moment by moment, to orient or to relate us to our surroundings in ways we might not otherwise have adopted. But here, we cannot possibly give a full account of all the remarks in Wittgenstein's works that have oriented us in this work. We can give only the merest hints.

7. As Wittgenstein (1953) puts it, this is a matter of "giving prominence to distinctions which our ordinary forms of language easily make us overlook" (no. 132). Such utterances as "stop," "look," "listen to this," "look at that" break routine ways of responding by pointing out features of the flow from within the flow (see no. 144).

8. ". . . don't think, but look!" (Wittgenstein, 1953, no. 66); "How hard I find it to see what is right in front of my eyes" (Wittgenstein, 1980, p. 39); "The aspects of things that are most important for us are hidden because of their simplicity and familiarity. (One is unable to notice something—because it is always before one's eyes.) The real foundations of his enquiry do not strike a man at all. Unless that fact has at some time struck him.—And this means; we fail to be struck by what, once seen, is most striking and most powerful" (1953, no. 129).

9. We have outlined these methods and their application in a number of articles elsewhere (Katz and Shotter, 1996a,b; Katz et al., 2000; Shotter and Katz, 1996, 1998).

REFERENCES

Bakhtin, M.M. (1981). *The Dialogical Imagination,* M. Holquist (Ed.), C. Emerson and M. Holquist (Trans.). Austin, TX: University of Texas Press.

Bakhtin, M.M. (1986). *Speech Genres and Other Late Essays.* Vern W. McGee (Trans.). Austin, TX: University of Texas Press.

Bakhtin, M.M. (1993). *Toward a Philosophy of the Act.* In M. Holquist (ed.), Vadim Lianpov (Trans.). Austin, TX: University of Texas Press.

Bateson, G. (1979). *Mind in Nature: A Necessary Unity.* London: E.P. Dutton.

Goffman, E. (1967). *Interaction Ritual.* Harmondsworth: Penguin.

Katz, A.M. (1991). Afterwords: Continuing the dialogue. In T. Andersen (ed.), *The Reflecting Team: Dialogues and Dialogues about Dialogues* (pp. 98-126). New York: Norton.

Katz, A.M., Conant, L., Inui, T., Baron, D., and Bor, D. (2000). A council of elders: Creating a community of care. *Social Science and Medicine* 50:851-860.

Katz, A.M. and Shotter, J. (1996a). Hearing the patient's "voice": Toward a social poetics in diagnostic interviews. *Social Science and Medicine* 46:919-931.

Katz, A.M. and Shotter, J. (1996b). Resonances from within the practice: Social poetics in a mentorship program. *Concepts and Transformations* 2:97-105.

Quine, W.O. (1953). Two dogmas of empiricism. In *From a Logical Point of View* (pp. 20-46). Cambridge, MA: Harvard University Press.

Sampson, E.E. (1993). *Celebrating the Other: A Dialogical Account of Human Nature.* New York and London: Harvester Wheatsheaf.

Shotter, J. and Katz, A.M. (1996). Articulating a practice from within the practice itself: Establishing formative dialogues by the use of a "social poetics." *Concepts and Transformations* 2:71-95.

Shotter, J. and Katz, A.M. (1998). "Living moments" in dialogical exchanges. *Human Systems* 9:81-93.

Voloshinov, V.N. (1986). *Marxism and the Philosophy of Language*. L. Matejka and I.R. Titunik (Trans.). Cambridge, MA: Harvard University Press.

Wittgenstein, L. (1953). *Philosophical Investigations*. Oxford: Blackwell.

Wittgenstein, L. (1980). *Remarks on the Philosophy of Psychology*, Volumes 1 and 2. Oxford: Blackwell.

Wittgenstein, L. (1981). *Zettel,* Second edition. G.E.M. Anscombe and G.H.V. Wright (Eds.). Oxford: Blackwell.

THERAPY:
"KNOWING-WITH"
IN THERAPEUTIC PRACTICE

Chapter 6

Relational Attunement: Internal and External Reflections on Harmonizing with Clients

Craig Smith

Power is not merely something we choose to take on or deny. It is invested in institutions and the roles we take on in society. As infinitely diverse in style as the relationships between therapists and the persons who consult them, it is the clients who come for "help," and it is the therapists who are therefore positioned as the "helpers." In this respect, therapists can be understood to be in a "power over" position, and without attention to these dynamics may impose ideas and practices even when they apparently negotiate the direction of the work with their clients.

Craig Smith is exquisitely sensitized to these issues, and has developed a number of ideas and practices which help him in at least approaching a relationship that is characterized by mutuality. He opens his chapter with reflections on four ways of knowing that he attends to as he strives to attune to the persons with whom he works. He then shares some ideas about how to approach therapeutic choice points in a way that enhances connection with clients.

To hold power over others means that the powerful is permitted a kind of short-cut through the complexity of human personality. He does not have to enter intuitively into the souls of the powerless, or to hear what they are saying in their many languages, including the language of silence.

Adrienne Rich, Of Woman Born[1]

I greet a returning client in the waiting room and we enter my office. She sinks into the now-familiar sofa and begins talking.[2] I immediately wonder how to participate with her. Does she want to make "small talk" while she reacclimates to being here again? Is she starting to give me important background material so I can understand the context of her pressing concerns? Is she a bit overwhelmed and unclear how to prioritize these concerns? Does she hope for something specific in return from me? Or should I perhaps remain silent right now because it is enough for her to have a safe place to think out loud and find her own clarity?

I often find myself silently asking these sorts of questions as I acclimate myself to clients. These client intentions are all valid ways of engaging with me. *But if I misapprehend what clients want from our time together at this particular moment, I may be out of sync and therefore unable to respond in a satisfying way.* For example, if the client is engaged in "small talk" about what happened during the week as a way to warm up to more important concerns, but I hear this as giving me background material for responding to some difficulty, we are at cross-purposes. If I begin giving advice in response to this material or investing my energy pursuing threads from this "warm-up," this can lead to difficulties. The client may begin experiencing self-doubt, wondering if I think there is something problematic in what she previously considered inconsequential; and I may begin getting frustrated when the client does not seem enthusiastic about my "good suggestions!"

It is challenging to position ourselves so that we minimize the risk of this type of disconnection and maximize the chance of exploring what is most meaningful for the client from moment to moment. However, rather than focusing on maintaining a strong connection with clients at all times, it seems more fitting to underscore the importance of clients sensing that therapists are making a sincere *effort* to have a resonant connection. Often this can have a "trial-and-error" flavor and can take pressure off therapists to have to "do it perfectly."

I will offer some ways of interacting in this chapter that have helped me in doing these things. I begin by discussing how important Tom Andersen's ideas of relational and bodily knowing have been in my harmonizing with clients and using more of myself in therapy. Next, I offer some reflections on how slowing myself down and being transparent with my thoughts have provided me with a more solid connection with clients. Then I discuss how eliciting clients' explicit expectations of me helps me to resonate more closely with them. Finally, I share some ways of asking for feedback, which is the way I like to end sessions.

FOUR WAYS OF KNOWING

When I was in graduate school, I felt bombarded by all of the different theoretical models. Each one seemed to have some merits, yet each one seemed to say, "Follow only me! The other models are suspect!" I was so eager to prove my mettle as a therapist that I clung to these models. These models were all traditional individual and systemic models (in contrast to postmodern/social constructionist approaches). Thus, clients were rarely presumed to be copartners in their own therapy and the therapist determined the focus of the work.

There were some advantages to becoming very familiar with these approaches. Many had some "tried-and-true" ways of assisting clients that were quite helpful and that I still utilize when appropriate. I could allay my anxiety about how to cope with ambiguous situations by remembering certain things to do. I could converse with my colleagues and with professors using professional lingo, which enhanced my credibility. Last and not least, I was able to pass my courses and eventually become licensed by familiarizing myself with this "conventional wisdom!"

There were also some disadvantages. I found that it was quite tempting to filter what the client said through the lenses these traditional theories espoused. Thus, when clients talked about their concerns, I often assumed I knew what they were "really" saying, according to whatever theoretical approach I was inhabiting. In addition, I often felt disconnected from clients. My "lifeline" was the theoretical lens rather than the person in front of me (Andersen, 1991). Furthermore, when I said things that did not fit for the client, the theory tended to blame the client for our missed connection (the client's defense mechanisms, cognitive distortion, resistance, and so on). Thus, I was invited to stay within this professional loop rather than to question my theoretical assumptions and to take the client more seriously.

In addition, I was so caught up with paying homage to the theoretical model I was inhabiting that I lost much of my organic sensibilities. While still responding spontaneously with friends and family, in the room with clients I robotically became an instrument or appendage of the theoretical model. Whatever inner reactions I had in response to what clients were saying that fell beyond what the *theory* said were relevant were obscured and dismissed. Consequently, much less of myself was available to clients.

When I first heard Tom Andersen talk about "four ways of knowing" (Andersen, 1996; Smith and Nylund, 1997, p. 171), I finally felt I had a way to make sense of my restricted inner responsivity. He spoke of rational knowing, technical knowing, relational knowing, and bodily knowing. Rational knowing includes things such as various theories of personality or theories of healthy systemic functioning. Technical knowing applies techniques or interventions derived from these theories. Relational knowing is the sort of sensibility that lets us know how to be with *this* particular person at *this* particular time in *this* particular context. Bodily knowing is the sort of understanding in which you have some sense in your body that something is significant but you are not sure to what this significance pertains.

Andersen suggests that all of these ways of knowing are important, but that, traditionally, rational and technical ways of knowing have predominated in the psychotherapy profession. These two ways have become so privileged that they determine what clinicians allow themselves to notice within the more intuitive relational and bodily modes. This speaks to my experience of having my natural sensibilities obscured or dismissed while with clients. He prefers to privilege the relational and bodily modes of knowing *while with clients,* but then *afterward* to reflect on rational or technical ways of thinking about what happened.

Andersen gave an example I enjoyed about relational knowing. He gave the analogy of being at home when a friend or loved one arrives. Your relational sensitivity allows you to tune in to where this other person might be at and to then respond accordingly. Do you see a furrowed brow and quickened steps? Perhaps the best thing might be to offer to make some hot chocolate for this person, or to simply let him or her be alone with his or her thoughts? Or perhaps you might ask if he or she would like to go for a walk, or to ask if it might be helpful to talk about what is happening (Andersen, 1996). We make these sorts of determinations all the time. We have a sense of what is called for in this particular context, space, and time. I think many people who enter the psychotherapy profession have heightened relational skills.

However, once I got into graduate school and into internships where I wanted to demonstrate my expertise and competence, it was very easy to lose touch with these natural, human sensibilities necessary for mutual dialogue. I wonder how my graduate experience might have been different if the "rational and technical" modalities were presented as offering provisional, general background information. How might things have been different if I had been encouraged to hold this information *lightly* so that my relational and bodily knowing could come forth more confidently and allow me to stay in the fullness and complexity of each particular moment in my evolving dialogue with clients?

Since I have allowed my relational and bodily knowing to play a greater part in my life with clients, I have felt much more alive and much more connected with them. After twenty years, I still look forward to witnessing and participating with clients. Each moment becomes yet another exciting and unpredictable opportunity to discover what seems to be called forth. "What is it I am sensing right now? Should I remain quiet or find a way to talk about my inner reactions? What seems to be most important right now for the client? What would they like me to do?" I find that asking myself these relational sorts of questions helps keep me focused. The more focused and connected I feel with the client, the more exciting, satisfying, and creative our time is together.

SLOWING MYSELF DOWN TO STAY CLOSER TO CLIENTS' MEANINGS

Another component in my "attunement dance" with clients is how closely I can resonate with or understand the clients' expressions. Once we start talking about pressing concerns, I find that I often may form premature assumptions about these concerns. In the ambiguity language constantly throws us into, I may "fill in the gaps" in ways that do not resonate with what the client wants to express.

I am particularly interested in how I can position myself or be present with clients to stay more closely within their meanings rather than to go off on premature tangents. Tom Andersen says, "I have to wait and see how the other responds to what I say or do before I say or do the next thing" (Andersen, 1995, p. 15).

My most resonant moments with clients often come when I slow myself down. Usually, the faster I try to work, the more chances I have to become out of sync. I become reactive rather than reflective, haphazard rather than resonant. I have found different ways to slow myself down.

My experience meditating has helped me tune in to what is happening inside and become less distracted by all the "signal noise." I would compare this to trying to look through choppy water versus looking through calm water in order to see what rests on the sand at the bottom. When I meditate, I am continually surprised at how clearly thoughts distill or solutions emerge to things I previously was in a quandary about. After meditating, I can sometimes carry some of this stillness and clearmindedness with me. Sometimes this self-awareness helps me see that I am feeling pressured to work too fast or to quickly come up with something really substantial for the client.

Sometimes I am able to remind myself not to jump to conclusions, to stay with the ambiguity and uncertainty for a bit. I advise myself to let my sails drift in the breeze rather than to succumb to rigidly steering. Frequently, if I am able to just listen openly in this way without locking on to one way of understanding, the client will spontaneously elaborate, giving enough details so I suddenly feel I am grasping how *the client* makes sense of this topic. This reminds me of times when I played baseball. While hitting, if I was impatient to make something happen, I would lunge at the ball and often not make solid contact with it. But if I had the presence of mind to relax and *let the ball come to me,* I had a much better chance of a good connection.

BEING TRANSPARENT

Sometimes just being aware of my habit to rush or reminding myself to stay with ambiguity is all I need to slow down and feel a more solid connection. If it is not, I may feel called to share the inner voices that lead me to this quickened pace. Perhaps my pressured quality has some connection to something I experience from the client? I can think of times when my desire to help has exceeded my nuanced understanding of what is involved. Part of me may sense the client's pain and urgency, and another part of me may not feel I have enough grasp of his or her context and unique background to be able to be of immediate help. If I am able to reflect on my inner voices, this may set the stage to openly share the dilemma these present for me with the client. I might say something such as, "I get the sense of how difficult things are for you right now, and I want very much to be useful to you. Instead of pre-maturely offering my perspective, I wonder if it might be OK right now to understand more of what is happening before getting into what to do about it?"

If I find that my own awareness of my inner experience or my self-reminders are not enough to feel reconnected with what the client is saying, I often share my thoughts as in the previous example. I find that this can create a mutually satisfying atmosphere. The client may be struck by my concern and by my risking such honesty. It may also give the client more encouragement to risk this honesty with me, with himself or herself, and with others.

Sometimes sharing my uncertainties out loud with clients takes the form of sharing competing perspectives or possible directions for discussion. I might say something such as, "Part of me is thinking that you might want to discuss how to talk with your daughter, but another part is thinking that you might be more pressured by what is happening at work . . . could you help me out here?" I also find that when I ask the client to slow down and elaborate in order to help me understand something that confuses me, he or she may become clearer about what he or she is trying to express as well.

More often than I would like to admit, I still may go ahead and make unwarranted assumptions and jump to conclusions about what the client wants. I may be so bewitched by my ideas about what is being said that I do not bother to really slow down and stay more with the moment-to-moment process. I may then get off on some tangent that holds little interest for the client. The client may be "going through the motions" with what I am saying, but with little spark or enthusiasm. The saving grace is that there usually are always opportunities to notice and repair this lack of good connection.

HOW CAN I HELP?

In twenty years of being with clients, I often find that talking explicitly about my participation can be quite beneficial. Some clients come in and have very distinct ideas about what they would like from me. Others are very murky about this. Some are somewhere in between. In addition to discussion topics, the client may also have some ideas about *how he or she would like me to engage* with these topics. Let us say a client comes in complaining of feeling depressed and saying he wants to talk about this topic. I might respond by asking, "Do you have any ideas about how I might be of help to you with this?"

The client may say, "Well, *you're* the professional . . . what are your ideas? What do you think would be best for me?" Or the client may not really have any clear ideas about my participation. Either of these possibilities is OK with me because I am trying to harmonize with clients. Knowing that this is where clients are, I no longer have to guess and I can respond accordingly.

When invited, many clients will say something more specific. Some might declare that they just want "a safe place to vent, be understood, and not be judged." Others may indicate they want specific advice or things to do about their depression. Some might say they want to know of good self-help books for their concerns. Still others may want to connect with groups of people facing similar issues. Some may wish to explore mixed feelings about medication.

I often like to follow up to these responses by asking for fuller elaboration. As discussed earlier, I like to stay as close as I can to fleshing-out implied meanings rather than make misguided assumptions about what is being said. I might say, "OK, you're saying you want 'a safe place to vent, be understood, and not be judged.' Could you say a bit more about this?" Or I could reply, "If this were to be such a place, how do you imagine this might help with your concern about being depressed?" I might say, "How would it be different if you were *not* feeling understood here or feeling judged?" I do not have a rote way of following up. My main goal is to try to get a fairly full sense of what the client means by these opening statements about my participation in order to maximize the chances that I can respond in a satisfying, harmonizing way, without making the client feel cornered or pressured to say more than he or she feels able to at that moment.

At times I may be uncomfortable with what the client expects of me and may need to negotiate with the client or possibly refer him or her elsewhere to get his or her needs met. If I am being asked to do things beyond my scope of practice, or to do things I do not feel prepared or qualified to give, I will share this. Thus, trying to attune myself with clients does not necessarily imply simple accommodation. Even though this chapter focuses on ways to attune with clients, I sometimes find that my retaining a divergent or contrasting viewpoint can be quite important. For example, a man who has physically abused his partner may inadvertently invite me to focus on ways to get his partner "more in line" rather than focus on ways he can become less violent and more responsible for his actions.

WAYS TO ASK FOR FEEDBACK

Given my preferences for staying closely connected to clients' moment-to-moment processes, I am continually asking myself or my clients how we are doing together. However, I do find that there are times and contexts in which I may do more or less of this. With new clients or clients with whom I feel particularly unsure of what they want from therapy, I often am more focused on these questions. I often rely on my sense of nonverbal feedback as well. If I feel as though clients are not particularly engrossed in what is being talked about, I may first get this sense from a blank expression, a monotone voice, or some other bodily indication. I do not want to assume I know the client's inner experience from these sorts of indications, but I do use these as gauges for getting more verbal feedback about our work together.

Sometimes I may get enthusiastic about a particular direction and get the sense that clients may not share my enthusiasm. I have seen some reauthoring therapists become very excited about a direction of inquiry and quickly ask clients something such as, "Is it OK if I ask you more questions about such and such?" Although I think the intent behind this question is quite well motivated, I do have some concerns about clients' degrees of freedom to respond honestly to this way of eliciting feedback. If clients see that we are indeed very excited about what we are talking about, that our voices are raised or our tone of voice has changed, and so on, they may feel it would be quite impolite to simply say something such as, "Actually, I'd rather talk about something else."

I think it is more likely that clients can respond more fully and honestly if they are presented with more open-ended sorts of feedback questions. This could sound something like, "I realize I'm quite enthusiastic about asking you more about this, but I'm not really sure where *you* are at. We could talk more about this, or we could talk more about x, y, or z. . . . What thoughts do you have about where to go from here?"

I often find it very helpful to leave room toward the last ten minutes or so to ask specific questions about our time together that day. Simply asking a general question such as, "How was today for you?" is likely to yield only a noninformative reply such as, "Fine." Thus I have found it most helpful to use specific yet open-ended questions. For example, "I realize we have talked about a variety of things today. What seemed to be a little more interesting or relevant?" I like to use "small" language ("a little more interesting") rather than asking for something more "substantial" ("what was really helpful today?"). I think that clients often need days or weeks to sort through these conversations before finding what has really impacted them, but they may well know immediately what was "interesting" or "relevant." Sometimes I may ask, "Was there anything we talked about today that might be worthy of playing with some more in the future?"

I also like to ask for the opposite. But, I do not want to make it too daunting for clients, because they generally do not want to insult us. Instead, I might ask something such as, "What sorts of things may have been a *little less* on the mark today, a *little bit less* central or relevant?"

CLOSING MOMENTS

I have shared some ways I try to harmonize or attune myself with clients. I discussed some of my professional journey and how important relational and bodily sensibilities have been for keeping me fresh, renewed, excited, and connected with clients. I have mentioned some ways I have found useful to keep myself more focused on clients' meaning making rather than be led astray by my premature assumptions. This frequently involves slowing myself down—doing a brief, internal check-in and/or outwardly sharing my internal process with clients. Even when I am bewitched by my own notions and become out of sync, I am inspired by the ever-present opportunity to notice and repair this disconnection.

I touched on ways to ask about my explicit participation, which provides an important ingredient beyond the content of what the client wants to discuss. And I concluded with some ways I have found useful for looking back on our meeting and looking ahead.

I hope there have been some aspects in this chapter that have been food for thought for you or perhaps have inspired you in some way. I feel as though our profession has given us the distinct privilege to listen to some of the most intimate and moving aspects of people's lives. It seems fitting that we continually ask ourselves how we can respond to this privilege in ways that honor our clients' voices, our own shifting sensibilities, and the mysterious and glorious dance of our interconnectedness.[3]

NOTES

1. I wish to thank Gretchen West for sharing this quote with me.

2. I arbitrarily will use female and male pronouns in this chapter.

3. A timely example of this interconnectedness is all the thoughtful feedback I received on earlier drafts of this chapter. I wish to express heartfelt appreciation to the following people who graciously spent their time and energy sharing their input and making this chapter more concise and rich: Lynne Rosen, Gretchen West, Peggy Sax, Todd Edwards, Debora Nylund, Dave Nylund, Lorraine Hedtke, Maggie Shelton, Abbe Slaney, Larry Laveman, Amy Huennekens, Lauren Eichen-Forsee, Mel Snyder, Stephanie Shulenberger, David Marsten, Wendy West, Jayne Reinhardt, Peter Rober, and especially David Paré.

REFERENCES

Andersen, T. (1991). Guidelines for practice. In Andersen, T. (Ed). *The reflecting team: Dialogues and dialogues about the dialogues* (pp. 42-67). New York: W. W. Norton.

Andersen, T. (1995). Reflecting processes; acts of informing and forming: You can borrow my eyes, but you must not take them away from me! In Friedman, S. (Ed). *The reflecting team in action: Collaborative practice in family therapy* (pp. 11-37). New York: Guilford.

Andersen, T. (1996). Dialogues and dialogues about the dialogues. Workshop presented at the California Family Studies Center/ Phillips Graduate Institute, Los Angeles.

Smith, C. and Nylund, D. (Eds.) (1997). *Narrative therapies with children and adolescents*. New York: Guilford.

SUGGESTED READINGS

Andersen, T. (1991). Guidelines for practice. In Andersen, T. (Ed.), *The reflecting team: Dialogues and dialogues about the dialogues* (pp. 42-67). New York: W. W. Norton.

Andersen, T. (1995). Reflecting processes; acts of informing and forming: You can borrow my eyes, but you must not take them away from me! In Friedman, S. (Ed.), *The reflecting team in action: Collaborative practice in family therapy* (pp. 11-37). New York: Guilford.

Anderson, H. (1993). On a roller coaster: A collaborative language systems approach to therapy. In Friedman, S. (Ed.), *The new language of change: Constructive collaboration in psychotherapy*. New York: Guilford.

Griffith, J.L. and Griffith, M.E. (1994). *The body speaks: Therapeutic dialogues for mind-body problems*. New York: Basic Books.

Chapter 7

Talking About "Knowing-With"
(Like a Team!)

Donald McMenamin

The professional literature most often turns to its theoretical arguments or disembodied empirical findings to assess the worth of therapeutic practices. Given that those practices invariably involve two or more persons in relationship, it is remarkable how little attention is given to deriving descriptive accounts from those persons themselves. A "knowing-with" orientation to evaluating practice encourages mutual exploration by therapists and the persons who consult them. For this chapter, school counselor Donald McMenamin chose not to *tell* what he does, but elected to *ask* instead. He met with students to get their account of what is helpful in his practice. The chapter takes the form of a multivoiced conversation in which McMenamin, his students, and friends speak of everything from room decor and process notes to body language and turns of phrase as they explore the ingredients of an inviting and helpful therapeutic approach.

This is an account of two conversations held at Hillcrest High School in Hamilton, New Zealand. The purpose of these conversations was to conduct research into a collaborative approach to counseling by hearing from young people about *their* experience of practice informed by a "knowing-with" metaphor. The input of four of those students forms the main body of this chapter.

The chapter is the product of two conversations. The initial conversation was taped and transcribed. I sent the transcript to a number of friends for their comments and questions.[1] Those comments and questions were the basis of a second conversation with my coresearchers Angeline Cox, Rachel Cranston, Sophie Jones, and Sue Schuitemaker.[2] The italicized text represents my voice, and the regular fonts the voices of the coresearchers. Questions in bold were posed by the outside readers and responses to them were blended into the final text here. We began by meeting in my office and I asked the question:

Why do you come here?

To talk to someone. It's easier to talk to someone who doesn't know me, judge me, tell me what to do, how to suss it out—they just listen. Also it's confidential—like with your mates you don't know who they'll tell. A guidance counselor helps you suss out yourself what you want to do.

[What is it that DM does that helps you do this?]

The picture thing—the way we draw pictures.
Tell me about that.
I don't know—the drawing out my problem like a picture—the problem resolves? You resolve it by the picture, but it's only a picture.
What is it about the picture? What does it do to you?
It's like my problem on paper. You see it in a different way and notice that it's not really that bad. Like it's bad, but not as bad as you think it is.
So one of the things that helps you suss it out is drawing the pictures. Can you think of other things that help you suss it out?
You tell us our options. Like the outcomes of different ways of sorting it out. Partly it is about being relaxing and stuff. Because you have got plants and things you just sit there relaxed and you can think about stuff.
I love having things to fiddle with! It's comforting. It helps you relieve stress or agitation or something.
So is there something about the environment?
Yeah, and it's like your face! You've just got a warm personality thingy. I always feel welcome when I come here. Like I've always felt welcome. Kind of nonjudging.
You can work through possible solutions. Instead of just one thing you can work on others, see what's best to do and get feedback on whether it's a good idea.
Have you had experience of speaking with someone who has tried to tell you what's wrong with you? What's that like?

I was in a custody battle—I had my own lawyer who was supposed to be for me. They listened to what I said and twisted it all to make me naughty—they had a pre-fixed judgment. It sucked because nothing could get through to them—they thought they were so much older and wiser than you and that you don't know what you are talking about. Actually, everyone is different and they do not know what they are talking about.

Can you contrast that with what happens here?

You [the student] are the boss. You are the one who knows the most about the person, and the person you are talking with does not know until you tell him or her what's going on. They've got to learn about you to help you solve your problems.

[How do you decide you can tell DM what's going on?]

You see your reaction to what's going on. And then it's "Oh sweet, I can say more!"

So you put a little bit out?

Yeah, and if it's bad, like your body language, we just close up again.

So there are things that I let you say and things that I don't? Do you notice that I shut you down on some things?

Yeah, like when we are dissing other people, and bitching. You're kind of like . . . [closed body shape].

Really? So there is something about my body language that says "No"?

Yeah.

So what is it that I do that gives you permission to say more?

Your face! And you go, "Yeah, yeah!" You give a sort of comfortable feeling about talking about it.

I'm interested in that, because in some ways I steer the conversation—you know? So do we always end up talking about the things you want to talk about? Or do I stop you sometimes from talking about the things you want to talk about? Like, who's in charge of the conversation really?

Both! Like we can stop. It depends really, because sometimes you want to know heaps about what we say, and sometimes we just drift on.

I'm interested in how much of what goes on in this room I control. I've got this idea that you guys are in charge of what we speak about.

But you tell me that sometimes I approve of some things and disapprove of other things.

Well, we have the idea; we bring the things. You make us think about it.

Do you ever feel shut down because of my body language?

It's happened before.

Is that a sort of trampling thing for you?

Yeah. I don't know about other people but . . .

What's different about going into a place with a pre-fixed idea and one where they've got to learn about you, where you are the boss?

You feel more in charge of what you are going through. You feel pretty powerless if someone is already judging you before you open your mouth, and already think they know about you before they do. But when you teach someone about you, you feel more in charge and you let them know what you want them to know. If you tell your friends what's going on with you, they can say "I know exactly how you feel." It's so annoying because no one knows exactly what you are feeling.

Have you experienced me asking questions to find out more about what you are feeling? What's that like?

It's good—you can get it all out. Sometimes it's hard. You don't know how to say it, or even if you want to. Sometimes it is easier to write or draw rather than talk.

Sometimes when you talk to people, like your parents, they can listen at the time but then bring it back up against you at a later time.

So you are not in charge of what happens with the information?

Yeah.

Do you experience yourself as in charge of the information here?

Yeah, because you can't use it for anything, because that is confidential.

I could use it for a diagnosis. I could use it to tell you what I think is wrong with you.

The thing is we don't really get a diagnosis here. We get feedback on what we are saying. We can find out what the problem is and how we feel about it—and change it if we want to. It's more like self-work.

Have you noticed that I think of your life as a story?

Yeah, you tell it as a story. You can picture yourself and your problem in a different way. You can see ways to avoid it. That time you talked about a problem as a tiger wandering around to eat you worked really well. I might not have understood it so well.

Instead of just "Oh man, I've got this massive problem," you put the problem as an obstacle in your story—the problem is just an obstacle to get over. It's not that big!

Sometimes I talk about problems as if they somehow had a life of their own.

The problem is the problem, the person is never the problem!

Exactly! The idea that there is nothing wrong with you—you are being harassed by a problem.

You realize you can actually change it. It's not always going to be with us—you can change it. Before this I didn't realize that.

[What happened in your talking with DM that helped you realize you could change it? Was there a particular moment?]

It says, "The problem is the problem, the person is never the problem," but the person is kind of like the feeding ground for the problem. And so, unless you stop feeding it, the problem is not going to go away. So you can't really say, "the person is never the problem."

Because there is a relationship between the person and the problem?

Yeah, the person isn't the problem.

But they're hooked into the problem in some way?

The first time I heard that "the problem is the problem" thing, I'd come here about a problem with my mum. It had got me to believe that I was the problem. I don't remember what you did, but you made me believe that I wasn't—that it was the situation.

And when that happened, what happened for you?

I felt like I could change it—because it wasn't me. It was just my relationship with my mum. And we started working on that relationship. When you hear, "The problem is the problem, the person is never the problem," it kind of tells you that you can change it. Because you can't always change yourself, but you can change some of the things that revolve around you. So it's like realizing that it's not you, but something around you, and you can change it.

Yeah. So that realizing that it's not you and "I can do something about it," that's the moment when change happens?

Yeah. That picture thing is important. And how you write down stuff. And you show it to us; you don't hide it.

Tell me about the showing it [notes taken] to you.

You just see everything you have said—so we know you are paying attention. And you say "Hold on a second!" so you can write something down. And that kind of gives you a little time to think. So it's not all just said.

It slows you down? Gives a kind of space?

Yeah. And when you read it you can add more things. You can think more. And also how you keep little files—you can remember things, and think, "Oh, I got through that."

How does it make you feel when you see you got over something? You can change something?

It gives you courage.

Does it?

You can go over the next hurdle.

So have you got more courage than you used to have?

Yeah!

If you could speak to counselors, what would you say to them about how to do their work?

The space you work in is important. Plants and relaxed, the vibe is comforting, a warm environment. You walk in and think, "This is sweet." The pictures are windows looking out of the room!

I reckon that people who are counselors need to have humor in it—it kind of lightens the whole thing up. You get deeper and deeper, then you have a little laugh. "Yeah, true!" It kind of makes you feel better. But you don't want to make a joke of the whole thing!

I'd say telling stories; the problem isn't attached to you, that problem rule—it's not you, it's the problem.

I'd want to say that not everyone is the same—each person they talk to is completely different. They deal with things in a completely different way. They should listen. I like just being listened to—not being told they know what it's like and what to do. They have no right to do that. It makes you feel better getting it all out, not being judged. You feel freer to say stuff. Don't butt in; let me speak.

I went to a counselor once who wrote stuff down but wouldn't show me it. She wrote out chores and stuff for me to do. She was solving the problems in my household, not my problems.

Do you notice that I take notes?

Yeah, but you take them down here (on the table) and they are in the open. And you take down what we say and the way we say it—like our own language, not yours. I know what they mean.

What's it like when you see notes being taken?

It's like "Did I actually say that?" I see it from a different point of view. It's like it's not from your mouth but from over there—you see it differently. And people are noticing what you are saying because you are taking it down. It's different seeing your thoughts on paper—you can see it instead of thinking about it.

I give you your file to look at when you first come in. What's that like?

It's got all this stuff in it from ages ago. Some of it does matter—they were problems but you have overtaken them. So it's like, "That was ages ago!" Sometimes I think, "Why did I come here for that?" You can look back over the times.

Sometimes I go through a person's file with him or her and ask, "What's useful or important in here?"

Because you could see a problem from ages ago and have a related one now—something a bit like that one—and think, "I got over it before," so it's kind of encouraging.

Sometimes it's embarrassing talking about stuff, but you need to.

So what's the role of the counselor when he or she senses you want to say something but are having difficulty with it?

It's tricky. Sometimes you want them to press it and sometimes not. You know by our body language. When it's clear that I don't want to talk about something and you say, "We'll leave that alone, eh?" it gives me a chance to sort of act myself on that—to decide for myself to talk or not to talk. Counselors just need to be on to it! You could try, "Do you mind if we talk about . . ." or "Do you want to . . ." They have got to have respect for you and for what you are going through. They have got to realize that it takes time—you don't get it all resolved in one little lesson. Ask "Is there anything specific you want to talk about?"

[This is really helpful and I'd love to know more about how you know the counselor has respect for you. Respect is a word that gets used a lot in counselor education and literature, but what do you think it means—how does it show itself?]

We just know you have respect for us, because when we walk into our classes our teacher doesn't know what we've just been talking to you about. And why would we keep coming back if we knew you didn't have respect for us?

And when you give us eye contact, and when we talk, you listen.
So these things make respect?
Yeah, like full concentration. And I hate it when people look at the clock to see how long you are taking!

Also, I like coming here and not being judged.
So that's about respect?
Yeah. If you talked to anyone else about it, you're going to be judged in some way. I suppose there is no way you could judge us—except in your mind.
Would you know if I did judge you in my mind?
Probably. Because when we came back you would treat us differently. Just the way you look at us. And if we came with others we would see you talk to them differently.
Do I talk to all people the same?
Pretty much.

And also you respect us by saying nothing at all in front of other people. Like when there are a few of us, and we might say, "I remember this," but you don't say anything, even when you know what we are talking about. And you don't ask about stuff you heard one to one when there is a group. Even if we are close friends.

Sometimes you start on something and it leads into something else. We can go off on tangents and end up in unexpected places!
Why is that good?
You can go wherever you like. "This is interesting!" Sometimes you forget what you were worried about, and when it comes up you can sort it. Like crossing a bridge when you come to it.
Is it weird to be giving advice to counselors?
It's like we are in the opposite scene. Usually we come here and talk about our stuff. It's weird to see you seeing it from a different perspective—us giving you advice. It's more of that power thing. We can tell you what's cool about the conversation without being in the conversation—without saying "Blah, blah, I've got a problem; by the way, I like the way you do that!"

I think it's cool because I bet counselors learn from other counselors. And now they can get advice from the people—it's because of us that they are counselors!
What advice would you give to people who are going to see a counselor?

I was too scared to come in when I was in Third Form (equivalent to U.S. grades 7 and 8)! I felt OK about going, but I felt new and like I needed to introduce myself. "Is my stuff significant enough to be here?"

I have some other questions and comments from people who read our first conversation. Can we respond to these?

[Just a comment—there is no shame in going to counseling.]

Sometimes there is shame. The teacher says, "OK, you can go to Guidance," and the whole class knows I was going to Guidance.

So is that a shaming feeling?

Sometimes people say, "Where were you?" "In Guidance." "Haha."

[Do you ever feel the counselor "tricked" you into thinking up a solution to a problem when it was really their idea?]

Yeah, I have at _____. I had this problem and the counselor just wrote up a chore list for me to do! And she sent me on my way. I thought "That wasn't really my problem, but . . . yeah."

[When did the students notice the shift had happened to them being a boss in the counseling room?]

When you gave us respect. Like you didn't look down on us. We're at the same level even though you are older than us. Also you can say "What do you want to talk about today?" or "What's the problem?" or "Who's first?"

You guys know my lines!

Yeah!

So there is something about those questions that makes you the boss. Yeah?

It's like we call the shots. It's what we say that matters. You talk in a way that joins us—undivided attention.

[DM is asking you about your ideas. Do you have some questions for him about how come he works in some of the ways you have identified as important?]

What are people going to learn from that?

It gives them a look into my head. Includes me in the picture.

I remember when you sometimes put a bit of humor into it. And I asked you, "Why do you always do that when it is such a serious matter?" I've forgotten your answer.

Yeah. I notice that too. But when you do do it, it doesn't seem to bother me. It usually makes me laugh!

I do do that, eh? There's a point where the tension gets to a certain level and I feel the need to lighten it up. Yeah. Is that OK?

Yeah. It's "as cool as."

It works all right?

Yeah. Sometimes when you talk to your friends they'll make a joke then change the subject right away.

That's about not paying attention?

Yeah.

But this is somehow about still paying attention.

Yeah. Showing the lighter side of what can be really bad.

What's it like for you when people walk in the door?

To me? It's exciting!

Why? You're weird!

I get a real buzz off seeing problems go away. I really enjoy it. It makes me feel like I am doing the thing I was made to do. So—maybe an artist gets the same buzz from drawing—I get that buzz off making things better. So, when people walk in the door, I've got a sense of expectancy. I expect good things to happen. And I am looking forward to that!

NOTES

We enjoyed talking about and writing about this stuff! It was neat when people read what we had said, and wrote back with questions and comments. The idea that our ideas are going into a book is really exciting! Also, we would be glad to hear back from people who read this and want to say what they think or what their experiences are.

Donald, Angeline, Rachel, Sophie, and Sue

1. The people who contributed comments and questions were Aileen Cheshire, Koichi Kunishige, Mary-Ellen McGarry, Hannah McMenamin, and Charmaine McMenamin.

2. In keeping with the title of this chapter, our work is aimed at working *with* students, families, and teachers to find ways that produce ourselves differently. Some

of our work in this area is found in the publication *Extending Narrative Therapy: A Collection of Practice-Based Papers* (1999), which was assembled by the Dulwich Centre in Adelaide, Australia. We are strongly influenced by the writings around narrative therapy including (besides the standard texts) the work of Aileen Cheshire and John Winslade (1997) published in *Narrative Therapy In Practice,* and Dorothea Lewis and Aileen Chesire (1995, 1998), "Talking Across the Generations" and "Taking the Hassle Out of School."

REFERENCES

Lewis, D. and Cheshire, A. (1995). Talking Across the Generations. *Dulwich Centre Newsletter,* 4:7-17.

Lewis, D. and Cheshire, A. (1998). Taking the Hassle Out of School. *Dulwich Centre Journal* 2 and 3:4-34.

White, C. and Denborough, D. (1999). *Extending Narrative Therapy: A Collection of Practice-Based Papers*. Dulwich Centre Publications: Adelaide, South Australia.

Winslade, J. and Cheshire, A. (1997). School Counseling in a Narrative Mode. In Monk, G., Winslade, J., Crocket, K., and Epston, D. (Eds.), *Narrative Therapy in Practice*. San Francisco: Jossey-Bass.

Chapter 8

A Room of Their Own

Jill C. Manning
Alan Parry

It takes more than earnest good intention to promote collaborative dialogue. Granting permission to another to share his or her concerns and hopes, as Craig Smith points out (in Chapter 6), is not as simple as reassuringly inviting him or her to speak "freely." In the context of family therapy, patterns and structures—not to mention family histories—hover over each spoken and unspoken word. Some stories are privileged; others are pushed to the margins.

This is certainly true in those cases when children come to sessions despite their stated preferences. In grappling with this dilemma in their work, Jill Manning and Alan Parry draw on the family therapy tradition of reflecting teams, with a twist, to make it possible for reluctant participants in sessions to listen and speak on something closer to their own terms. This chapter describes the development of this clinical innovation and poses some suggestions for alternate ways to literally "create space" for otherwise silent family members to share their experiences.

I thought of the organ booming in the chapel and of the shut doors of the library; and I thought how unpleasant it is to be locked out; and I thought how it is worse perhaps to be locked in.

Virginia Woolf, *A Room of One's Own*

A common predicament within family therapy practice is the inclusion of a hostile child or adolescent who is present against his or her will, yet whose participation seems necessary for family therapy to proceed. In this chapter, an intervention that has been found helpful in reversing the self-exclusion of the angry youth will be presented. This approach offers the young person an opportunity to contribute in a noncoercive way at the same time addressing the implicit (and possibly explicit) coercion that may have been involved in getting the youth to therapy in the first place.

Often, parental coercion is evident when a child is pressured to participate despite having made his or her reluctance, even refusal, to comply very clear. At times, the youth's protests may escalate to the point where the therapist and the beleaguered parents are ready to throw in the proverbial towel and excuse one party from the therapeutic process or propose therapy in tandem. With each of these alternatives, however, the richness of working directly with family interactional patterns is mitigated.

The authors have struggled with this predicament on several occasions and have become increasingly curious about alternative ways of dealing with this therapeutic dilemma. Options that maintain the therapists' integrity toward postmodern assumptions regarding nonimposition, all the while remaining systemic, have been of particular interest.

INITIAL FORMULATION AND APPLICATION OF THE INTERVENTION

The intervention highlighted in this chapter sprang out of a particularly challenging family therapy session in which all parties, including the two therapists present, were feeling stuck and unsure of how best to proceed toward a therapeutic end. The first author, Jill, who at the time was a cotherapist in the aforementioned session, became increasingly aware of the eldest son's reactivity toward his parents as the session progressed. The son's reactivity manifested itself through verbal maliciousness, profanity, and self-imposed silence. Subsequently, the parents were invited into taking a more rigid and closed stance, thereby perpetuating the relational violence that had brought the family to therapy in the first place.

The therapists wrestled with the dilemma of how best to capitalize on the process occurring in the room to bring forth a therapeutic shift. It was tempting to invite the parents or the youth to leave the room and proceed with the session in a more peaceful manner. Both therapists, however, were keenly aware of the deficit this would create in the conversation about family dynamics, not to mention the risk of alienating one or both parties from the therapeutic process.

Having the reflecting team process in mind, and being aware that the family and the therapists felt stuck, Jill became curious about the effects of modifying the traditional reflecting team format and having the unruly child join her in the adjacent observation room to view the rest of the session between the parents and the other therapist. Taking Dr. Tom Andersen's (1987) viewpoint that a stuck system is one in which there are too many repeating samenesses and too few differences, introducing a variation of the reflecting team process was viewed as a possible way to counter the sense of being stuck, generate alternate meanings, and circumvent an escalating situation in a nonviolent manner. Jill was especially curious about what would happen if both she and the reactive youth were able to benefit from the reflecting process in a collaborative way. In short, expanding the therapeutic space to include the reflecting team room was viewed as a means to temporarily counter the violent practices emerging in the session while preserving the family therapy process.

Once the idea had come into focus, the next step was introducing it in a manner, and at a time, that it would most likely be received. During a lengthy period of silence in the session, Jill figured that the session had been stalled to a such a degree that suggesting something new would likely be welcomed as long as it was an "appropriately different" idea, meaning it included enough samenesses from the preceding conversation so as not make the family system experience more anxiety, but enough difference to be a catalyst for movement (Andersen, 1987).

Jill opened the idea by stating, "I have an idea. I am not sure what will happen by introducing this idea, but I would be curious about where it could take us." At this point the nonverbal cues in the room encouraged Jill to continue in sharing her idea. "Aaron [not the client's real name], see this screen here?" Jill pointed toward the adjacent venetian blind covering the two-way mirror, and Aaron looked toward the covering. "This blind covers a two-way mirror. Behind it there is a small room where people can go to view what goes on in here and then share their ideas or viewpoints about what they have seen. When there are people in there, they can hear and see what happens because of special microphones and light switches. I am wondering if you would like to join me back there and watch the rest of the session between your parents and the therapist?" Aaron, who had been silent for some time now, gave a shrug of agreement and started to move toward the door. Aaron's parents and the other therapist were visibly surprised with his positive reaction and proceeded to prepare the room for observation.

As soon as Aaron and Jill were outside of the room and were walking around to the reflecting team room, Jill explained that she and Aaron would simply observe the rest of the session, and that at the end of the session they could decide if they wanted to offer a reflection. The reflection, as it was explained, could consist of a comment, observation, or question by one or both of them. It was made clear to Aaron that he would have a choice about his involvement and that his wish to remain a silent observer would be respected if that was his preference.

Once settled in the reflecting room, Jill turned off the lights, turned on the microphone, and tapped on the window to notify the parents and the other therapist that they were ready to begin observing. The session proceeded, and Jill and Aaron sat casually watching. Jill subtly but consciously mimicked Aaron's posture to foster a sense of joining with him as they watched the session together. Jill made every effort to take a nonexpert stance with Aaron in order to validate the knowledge and expertise he had about his family and to contrast the power differentials in the interview room that had heightened his reactivity just moments ago.

To Jill's amazement, within minutes of being in the room of his own, as it were, Aaron began to make comments, offer opinions, and share feelings concerning the family predicament and the unfolding interview. His initial comments were in the form of a monologue; Jill continued to observe the interview. Within fifteen minutes, however, Aaron and Jill were engaged in a lively dialogue about what was happening in the interview room. Jill strived to maintain a stance of curiosity during this conversation. Questions such as, "What do you make of that, Aaron?" and "What is your theory on that?" and "From your experience in this family, what would you say are some of the important changes that would need to be made for people to get along better?" were examples of the kinds of questions that punctuated the dialogue and Aaron's input.

By the end of the session, the previously agitated youth had opened up in an unprecedented way and had prepared several questions and comments that were then relayed to the interview room through the microphones and two-way mirror. To some degree, it is believed by Jill that the opportunity to use audio equipment was intriguing and "appropriately different" in and of itself to solicit a reflection from a thirteen-year-old boy. Aaron's reflection allowed the therapists and parents an opportunity to learn about the youth's ideas about the family and possible solutions to resolve the conflict. The session ended on a respectful and hopeful note, an atmosphere in sharp contrast to the first half of the interview.

Essentially, the shift in interview format afforded Aaron the chance to get out from under the therapeutic and parental gaze, not to mention the hot seat of being questioned as the "problem child." Aaron's desire for exclusion and inclusion was also simultaneously honored and his expertise and feedback were then accessed. Needless to say, Aaron's contribution added a much-needed dimension and perspective to the layered family and therapeutic knowledge, fostering an atmosphere of collaboration and movement that had not been present prior to this intervention.

Looking back, it is the authors' opinion that creating an atmosphere of "no expectations" and creating space, literally and figuratively, for the existence of this family's "other" child, afforded Aaron the safety and sense of empowerment to become openly engaged in the therapeutic process. His openness, it should be noted, was evident almost immediately after leaving the therapy room and first manifested itself in a more relaxed body posture and demeanor.

SUBSEQUENT APPLICATIONS
OF THE INTERVENTION

Curious about how this approach could be applied with other families, the authors began introducing it to a variety of families who presented with children or adolescents in similar stances of noncompliance or hostility. In all cases thus far, positive results have ensued. To date, the approach has been introduced and set up in like fashion to the initial application. Results have included children being open to collaborating on reflections, children agreeing to join the next therapy session with all family members in the same room, children offering valuable narratives about family life and possible solutions that had not been heard or previously considered, and parents acknowledging how their own gaze had been closing space for their child.

In all cases, the approach has been introduced when the interview has stalled due to reactivity or relational violence occurring in the session. So far, the format has not required lengthy explanation for the youth or parents to try it because it has been introduced when family members are frustrated or are unsure of how to proceed. In other words, the intervention has been introduced with a tentative and enthusiastic tone when the sentiment "what have we got to lose?" pervades.

If, however, one or all parties were less responsive to the idea, it could be explained as an opportunity for a member of the family to listen to other family members in a new way, and for those in the interview to experience being audienced in a new way by the child. The novelty of the situation, it could be explained, holds the possibility of generating fresh insight, alternate meanings, and solutions previously not thought of while engaged in the joint interview process. The explanation could continue by stating that often when people are in a family meeting, they are so preoccupied with what they are going to say next that they miss out on hearing and learning valuable information about the others' experience. The proposed shift in format allows people to audience one another in a way that takes the pressure to have to immediately respond off and allows a more relaxed and open atmosphere wherein people can use their expertise and voice in new ways.

THEORETICAL POSSIBILITIES: SPACE, STATUS, AND THE STRUGGLE FOR RECOGNITION

From a theoretical standpoint, three key points provide a framework for understanding why this approach has facilitated positive results. These theoretical speculations include the opening of physical and psychological space, the influence of status and power differentials within family systems, and the honoring of the youth's struggle for recognition and voice.

Opening Space

Introducing the reflecting-team room into the session literally expands the physical and psychological space in which people can generate, hear, exchange, and reflect upon alternate meanings to problematic narratives. This kind of exchange produces what J. L. Bogdan referred to as an ecology of ideas, and subsequently thickens an ongoing process of change and adaptation (Andersen, 1987).

From a physical point of view, the therapeutic arena is expanded by virtue of adding an adjoining room to the interview space. The physical space fosters a sense of safety due to the improbability of violent confrontation. The subsequent decrease in anxiety liberates people to listen more attentively to others, not to mention their own thoughts.

From a psychological standpoint, there is an opening of space wherein the youth can reclaim ownership over the degree to which he or she will participate, all the while being connected in a meaningful way to the family therapy process. Similarly to the way a spontaneous inhalation occurs when the physical body is stretched, the stretched therapeutic space is conducive to psychological inhalation, and the assimilation of ideas and meanings that could not be received while in an anxious, and closed state (Friedman, 1995, p. 14).

Status and the Struggle for Recognition and Voice

Upon relaying the initial intervention and its positive result to Dr. Alan Parry, who at the time was Jill's clinical supervisor, two closely related themes of considerable interest to him immediately came to mind: (1) the question of status and the struggle for recognition within family systems, and (2) the issue of how family members give to and gain from one another a voice of their own.

Parry has long been influenced (1973, 1996) by Hegel's dialectic position that human interactions involve a struggle for recognition, during which, in the effort to reduce anxiety, one subordinates to another to obtain such recognition as that allows, taking what Hegel calls the "slave" position to the extent that the other refuses to yield the dominant or controlling position of the "master." Perhaps in Hegel's world the struggle for recognition did invariably resolve itself in such a manner. Probably in "rights"-oriented societies, such as our own, the struggle is not so simply relinquished but goes on interminably. Today, fewer settle for the slave position, and most long for relationships of mutual recognition.

We suspect that the struggle for recognition is an inescapable feature of family life. Parents and children each seek recognition from the other and neither yields in its pursuit. Children are enabled to develop a voice of their own when and to the extent that they are given status or recognition within the family by being listened to and having their words and opinions taken seriously. To the extent that a child fails to experience himself or herself as being heard he or she is apt to seek recognition by at least being noticed. Disruption and defiance in the pursuit of recognition tends to have the unfortunate effect that the parents either yield and assume the slave position to the child, who in turn takes the master position of inappropriate domination, or else the parents attempt to obtain what they consider to be their due recognition through coercive means which invariably fail. The child, in turn, tends then to escalate in his or her determined struggle for recognition.

When such children are designated as nothing but troublesome characters in their parents' version of the family story, this becomes the best form of recognition available to them. They are then characterized in a thinly plotted way by a pathologizing label that becomes the only role available within the family drama for them to gain the recognition they crave. Left with only that choice, in accordance with White's (1986) reminder of Bateson's dictum that people act as they do because they are constrained from acting otherwise, the entire family finds itself locked in a room from which they do not know how to escape. Parents seek dominance status in the family largely through language: "Now you do just as I say!" Children also vie for dominance but through enactment in the form of relentless demands. The trip to the therapist is a visit to a place where the parents' preferred medium of language is expected to prevail. They will explain to the therapist, a fellow adult, what they are being forced to contend with so that the therapist can give the offending behavior the appropriate subordinate label. Jill's intervention addresses those situations in which the child refuses to cooperate, but instead succeeds in dominating the situation by actions rather than words.

In the case of Aaron, by offering to take him out of the "locked" room and bringing him to a room of his own, he was given new status and a different kind of recognition. He was taken from a marginalized position in the family and suddenly given a privileged one. It is vitally important that anyone have a room of one's own in which to enact a new position. When that takes place it is remarkable how rapid change can be. The situation with Aaron suggests just how strong the yearning for recognition is in us all. It also suggests that, given the choice and the chance, a child is more likely to embrace recognition that is affirming and confirming over the coercive kind that he or she knows has not been freely given.

ALTERNATIVE APPLICATIONS

The authors are aware of the luxury afforded them in having access to facilities that lend themselves to shifts in interview format. For the majority of therapy sessions, however, clinicians may not have the benefit of having reflecting rooms or the equipment necessary to duplicate the intervention described. Alternatives to this kind of intervention, however, may be used to achieve equivalent results.

For example, if only one room is available, chairs could be arranged so that one therapist and the parents are on one side of the room and the cotherapist and child are sitting together in a different part of the room. With everyone in the same room, the degree of tandem conversation would need to change, but all parties would be able to benefit from the reflecting process.

For situations in which only one therapist is working with a family, the therapist may continue the session with the parents and have the youth sit apart from the group to listen as he or she sees fit. When appropriate, the therapist could then join the youth in his or her area of the room, and invite the parents to sit back and observe while the therapist attempts to engage with the youth and collaborate on reflections about the interview's content and process.

Aside from the logistics of the intervention, one must also consider the varying degrees of client readiness for and acceptance of such approaches. Depending upon how open the person being invited behind the mirror is, the therapist could decide to engage more directly with the client in a collaborative conversation about how the session has progressed thus far and what needs to change for therapy to continue in a nonviolent manner, pausing briefly now and again to listen and comment on what is being said in the main interview room.

In more volatile situations, the therapist and client could choose to remain silent for the duration of the reflecting room time and focus exclusively on listening to the session in the interview room, finishing the session with a more traditional reflection. The client may also choose not to be involved in a reflection of any kind, at which point the therapist could either speak briefly about his or her own experience or invite the client to comment during the following session.

The intervention outlined in this chapter was initially an attempt to circumvent a hostile family situation from escalating. After discussing the unexpected results more in depth and being curious about how it would work with other families, the authors came to a more mindful awareness of why the approach was bringing forth positive results. The intervention is believed to facilitate positive results because it opens physical and psychological space wherein family members may enact different status positions in relation to one another and the struggle for recognition within the family is shifted in an appropriately different way. In essence, the intervention allowed for the richness of family therapy to be harnessed while at the same time shifting the format enough to counteract the repeated samenesses occurring in the room. This shift in format enabled the therapists to overcome the impasse as well as the temptation to exclude a member of the family temporarily. This intervention was particularly valued for its respectful and nonimpositional stance. This stance reinforced for the authors the idea that a struggle for recognition is a feature of family life and that when children are provided space and opportunity to develop a voice of their own, they are less inclined to seek recognition through domination.

REFERENCES

Andersen, T. (1987). The reflecting team: Dialogue and meta-dialogue in clinical work. *Family Process* 26:415-428.

Friedman, S. (Ed.) (1995). *The reflecting team in action: Collaborative practice in family therapy*. New York: Guilford Press.

Parry, A. (1973). "The triumph of Eros: The prospects for community after Freud." Unpublished doctoral dissertation, Graduate Theological Union, Berkeley, CA.

Parry, A. (1996). Story enactments. *Context: A news magazine of family therapy and systemic practice* 28:20-24.

White, M. (1986). Negative explanation, restraint and double description: A template for family therapy. *Family Process* 25:169-184.

SUGGESTED READINGS

Berne, E. (1964). *Games people play.* New York: Grove Press.

Berne, E. (1972). *What do you say after you've said hello? The psychology of human destiny.* New York: Grove Press.

Johnstone, K. (1982). *Impro: Improvisation and the theater.* London: Methuen.

Johnstone, K. (1999). *Impro for storytellers.* New York: Routledge.

Parry, A. and Doan, R.E. (1994). *Story re-visions: Narrative therapy in the postmodern world.* New York: Guilford Press.

Chapter 9

Young People and Adults in a Team Against Harassment: Bringing Forth Student Knowledge and Skill

Aileen Cheshire
Dorothea Lewis
The Anti-Harassment Team

There is a certain paradox in encouraging youth to interact in responsible and accountable ways by legislating their actions through the imposition of adult-generated guidelines. Why should young men and women rely on their own judgment when those in authority legislate their actions from the top down? In their work with youth in Auckland, New Zealand, Aileen Cheshire and Dorothea Lewis resist the temptation to slip into a "knowing-that," choosing instead to forge a response to harassment *with* their students.

That collaborative spirit extends to the composition of this chapter, which was co-authored with the Anti-Harassment Team at Selwyn College. The chapter recounts the development of a peer mediation program that is gaining attention on both sides of the equator. Interestingly, the authors' attention turns not to the didactic content of the "training," but to the manner in which school counselors and the team have managed to create a collaborative relationship that pays true homage to the students' judgment and abilities.

The Anti-Harassment Team is a group of twenty-four young people, aged fifteen to eighteen, at Selwyn College in Auckland, New Zealand, who are involved in peer mediation, offering young people a possibility of resolving conflicts peacefully without adult intervention.[1] The team does not claim to have eliminated the problem of harassment or bullying, but there is now a culture at the school in which students request help with conflicts early on and talk to one another in mediation in a process where everyone has an equal voice.

Issues brought to the team range from friendship difficulties and the effects of gossip, rumor, and teasing to serious racial and sexual harassment. The team's stand against harassment and violence in the school includes classroom workshops that make visible the practices and power of harassment. Once harassment is named and exposed, and ways are found to speak and act against it, it becomes a far less acceptable part of school life. It has become commonplace for the team to meet new junior students whose lives have been made miserable by bullying practices during their years of primary schooling, who discover once they come to Selwyn College that there are alternatives to having to put up with this. Mediation offers a possibility for the young person to have a voice and agency in sorting out the problem in a way he or she has never experienced before. Many of them have experienced adults' well-meaning attempts to impose solutions that have left them feeling in some way deficient or lacking in capabilities.

In a school setting it is often the adults who are positioned as holding expert knowledge (Winslade and Monk, 1999). Our purpose in this chapter is to explore how the students of the Anti-Harassment Team have come to be "experts" in mediation and in working against peer harassment. In doing so, we recognize that there are many different voices to be heard. There are our adult voices as counselors who have worked with the team since its beginnings. We are therapists who are on the staff of the school. Then there are the voices of past team members whose knowledge has been incorporated into the team. Within the current team there are voices of experience that speak of knowledge developed in the two or three years of belonging to the team, and there are the voices of those new to the team who bring a different and sometimes challenging perspective on the team and of practices of harassment in the school. Our dilemma here is how to allow these many different voices to be heard.

Yet it is precisely finding ways to privilege the voices of young people that has led to the successful practice of the team. For this reason this chapter is not a blueprint of how to run a peer mediation program (Lewis and Cheshire, 1998). Rather, it is an exploration in writing of the relationships and the ideas which have led to a student-centered service that is used regularly and effectively by students in the school. The writing has direct quotations taken from transcripts of tape-recorded conversations with the students, which became the basis of further discussion.

When we were invited to write this chapter as a collaboration between the adult counselors and the young people of the team, as adults we were uneasy about possible restraints on the team's voices, which would limit or silence their contributions. In the first meeting to discuss the invitation we declared this unease. The process began with a wide-ranging discussion in response to the idea of "working with." The transcript of this provided key ideas which were then explored more fully in individual or small groups. The team reviewed the first rough draft with two counseling interns facilitating the discussion rather than one of us, in case our presence in some way inhibited the discussion.

WORKING AS ADULTS WITH A TEAM OF YOUNG PEOPLE

As counselors in a school we have both chosen a stance that challenges conventional power relationships between adults and young people. This is not about techniques or methods. It is about a way of being with people—a relational stance (Bird, 2000), in which we try to work alongside students as allies. We have become aware over the nine years of the team's work that the effectiveness of their work is in some measure due to this culture of collaboration, in that it has led to a genuinely student-centered service.

Sebastian reflects on how we have developed the relationship: "You don't organize how to treat us—it's just a relationship you're in. It's not a phony relationship. You're not like teachers telling us what to do all the time. You give us the freedom to develop our own ideas and treat us as individuals."

Harriet continues, "So you classify our ideas I suppose as just the same as your ideas. Like a lot of the processes we go through during the year for the workshops and the symposiums you actually rely on our ideas—or you seem to! You give us very broad boundaries for the workshops and then let us organize what we think will work best. So we work within those boundaries or the framework. And that makes us feel like we are important, like our ideas count."

Lisa adds, "Dorothea and Aileen are tentative about giving their ideas, but they will always suggest things if you ask them."

Yet we are also aware that we bring knowledge to this work—knowledge that comes from working with the many students who have been in the team over nine years and knowledge that comes from our counseling practice. We carry these knowledges but hold the firm belief that they are neither fixed nor static. And there is much that we do not know. So, how do we create experiences that will enable different knowledges to be brought forth? How do we avoid privileging what we know over the knowledge the team brings? How do we know *and* not know? We are drawn to Johnella Bird's description of therapists as "discoverers of knowledge" (Bird, 2000).

Ezra, who has now left school, describes this relationship with knowledge: "So I think there are different areas of knowledge. Aileen and Dorothea's from their counseling work and the team members from doing the mediation work and knowing what is effective. What's really important is the team has knowledge about establishing links with young people which comes from knowing about young people's cultures and what is happening for them. The adult knowledge comes from a different sort of experience—like knowing how to discover things with asking questions."

In a group discussion facilitated by two counseling interns, students in the team responded to questions (in italics) about the relationship between Aileen and Dorothea as adults and the student team members: *How do you know you are being treated with respect?*

"Seeing them talk to each other and then seeing the way they talk to us is the indicator."

Is the quality of the relationship important in defeating harassment?

"The relationship between us and Dorothea and Aileen is reflected in how we do mediations. If it was more of a student-teacher thing, I don't think people would be as open as they are to us because we . . . we've been given the chance to develop and grow."

What if it was a top-down relationship?

"We probably would take the power imbalance into a mediation. They encourage joint exploration and you can take that interest into a mediation with you."

Many students spoke of the pride and satisfaction they gain from doing work they have a strong commitment to (Bruell, Gatward, and

Salesa, 1999). The team does not do this work because they are told to or to please the adults. Sebastian sums this up: "We don't try to make Dorothea and Aileen happy. It's 'I've solved the problem and I'm happy about that.'"

STEPPING BACK AS ADULTS

When we first began working with the students of the team we "took on" mediating what we saw as more difficult situations. Usually these were situations that involved physical violence, in which there was some concern for safety in the mediation. There was an unspoken assumption that adults were more able mediators and that physical violence made mediation more difficult. We were positioned as the mediation experts and the student members of the team as less capable because of their age. Supporting these assumptions was the idea that adults have expert knowledge in controlling young people. In practice the school management, who referred students for mediation directly to us whenever a so-called difficult situation erupted, reinforced our expert position.

These assumptions were put under the spotlight when a fifteen-year-old mediator calmly stopped a mediation when one of the fourteen-year-old participants pulled a knife. Jody, the mediator, immediately turned to the school management for support and the fourteen-year-old was suspended. The suspension stipulated that another mediation take place before the student could come back to class. In talking about her experience afterward, Jody was certain that she wanted to finish the mediation process. Despite a strong request from the school management that one of the counselors conduct the mediation, we supported Jody to finish what she had begun. Our thinking at the time was clear. If we as adults had stepped in and taken over from Jody we would have undermined her credibility. The mediation was successfully resolved and both parties developed a greater understanding of each other. In looking back Jody said that continuing this mediation was a marking point in her recognizing the abilities she had as a mediator.

In consulting with mediators from another school who were wondering why their mediation team had little work, we wondered if an important difference in that school was that the counselors had continued to do the more "difficult" mediations. The teacher in charge of the mediation team was also sitting in on mediations to support the student mediators. This was a shock to us, as we have from the beginning of this work shown that our support means we are available but not physically present in mediations. To be so would undermine the authority of the mediator and have the potential to silence or shape the conversation between peers. Our learning continues to be about who defines support and what forms it takes.

It is interesting to note that Selwyn College supports the work of the team by allowing mediations to take place during class time, without an adult present. This has developed from a belief that effective learning cannot happen if students are preoccupied with trouble or fear.

DISCOVERING STUDENT KNOWLEDGE

So what has led us to invent and reinvent ways of structuring our so-called training so that young people become discoverers of knowledge rather than learners from us as adults? We can identify some key moments in this development. Having started our mediation training together when we employed a trainer to come to the school in 1993, we assumed the traditional teacher approach of staying one step ahead of the students in teaching them. This position was challenged by a realization, when transcribing a tape of a mediation for a manual we were writing, that the student mediator had a level of expertise that was beyond ours.

Ezra explains his experiences of the growing recognition of student knowledge: "In the beginning we did get an outside mediator in who was really directive in his teaching style. I enjoyed that, as it took my thinking another step further. But it says something for the way knowledge is developed in the team, that he only came in at the beginning because what he taught us was adapted and passed on in a way that people new to the team could relate to. It's like we made that knowledge ours."

The mediation process the team has developed does not fit neatly into any specific mediation model (Winslade and Monk, 2000). It is the accumulation of ten years' "indigenous knowledge." Although this knowledge is accumulated and developed throughout the year, it is at a three-day training camp that team knowledge is specifically highlighted and passed on.

PASSING ON STUDENT MEDIATION KNOWLEDGE

Anton reflects, "In the first two years I was on the team, the knowledge about mediations seemed to be coming from Dorothea and Aileen or from Peter Stallworthy, the mediator brought in to teach the team. I think there was a big shift when Aileen and Dorothea stopped doing the more difficult mediations. That meant we were seen as having ability. At the same time in training there was a shift to the team members demonstrating, which really brought out the ability and knowledge in the team. That year at camp, Esther mediated a roleplay mediation around racial harassment which got very real and everyone got involved. When we saw Esther working in that tense situation, we had great respect for what she could do. And she was one of us."

The training camp involves the team, Dorothea, and Aileen living together away from school for three days, working together to develop knowledge and ability as we include new members. An example of an exercise at last year's camp was to ask a senior team member to be the mediator, and two other students to concoct a realistic scenario in which they could play the roles of two people coming to a mediation. The rest of the team observed the mediation. As the mediation ran its course, Aileen wrote all the questions the mediator asked on the whiteboard. Once it finished, Dorothea asked the mediator to reflect on what had happened in the course of the mediation and asked the two role-players to speak about what they had experienced. After a general reflection, the three were asked to look at the progression of the mediation as shown by the listed questions. They could then comment on which questions had been important, useful, and helpful from each of their standpoints. The rest of the team could then ask questions of the mediator such as "What made you choose that question then?" or to the role-players, "What was the effect on you when he asked. . .?" The team seemed very involved and focused for the ninety minutes this exercise took, and many of them chose to stay and write notes when it was all finished.

Another activity the team has identified as being useful in training is a "caucusing" mediation. We ask for volunteers for the roles of mediator and participants. The team sits in a circle around the mediation. As it unfolds, one of us acts as a sociodrama director, freezing the action, asking observers to comment and take a position on what they see. The observing team members identify with a particular role and are asked to join in, sitting behind the role player. The aim is to have the full team involved. Sometimes we will set up an observer group who will report back at the end. When the action is frozen, each role group, as they have become, can consult and caucus. Sometimes this can lead to intense feelings of involvement. Students tell us this gives them the experience of sitting in the different positions within a mediation, leading to an understanding of different points of view. The activity finishes with a debriefing of each group.

Anton: "I remember knowing I had ability and knew about mediations when I was asked to demonstrate what I knew. That's a great confidence builder—teaching or demonstrating. But training within the team also builds a strong group culture, as it builds confidence in the effectiveness of the team. I think when the team is really a team, when people feel supported and privileged to belong, then that boosts effectiveness."

Sophie and Keri, who joined the Team recently, reflect on camp: "I learned most working in small groups because we were given the chance to have a go. To begin with I thought doing a mediation was going to be real easy, but then I had a go and fell apart! But from then on it made more sense and I could understand what things were useful and why. Having more experienced team members sitting with me as I had a go was great. They gave me so much support, giving me ideas to try, possible questions to ask and just supporting me to try. No one said, 'don't do it that way,' but they'd say, 'You could try this . . . or maybe this.' So nothing was forced on you. I think the thing about learning from other team members is that you can share your uncertainties more easily with them—at the beginning anyway.

What seems important about mediations is that I learned there is no right or wrong way to do things. So that leads to the acceptance of different ways of getting to the same place. I felt I could really have my own style."

We have come to realize the importance of students bringing their own style within the structure of a formal mediation. Sometimes this can leave space for difference in cultural approaches. For example, Moana, one of the mediators who describes herself as coming from the Cook Islands, concludes her mediations with an appropriate song.

When asked about the most helpful learning situations on camp, Isaac, new to the team, thought: "Watching a past team member mediate on video with the video being stopped at significant points made me really think, 'What would I be saying? If I asked that question what direction would the mediation take? What was the idea behind my question?' That was a really helpful exercise. Seeing Lewis mediate instead of an adult made a big difference. You two [Aileen and Dorothea] have degrees in counseling and lots of counseling experience, but watching one of us mediate makes me realize, 'if he can do it I can do it.' It felt more achievable. The way I see you working as adults with us is that you set up exercises or ideas and you might not know exactly what is going to happen, but you let us do it and that's really important. It's like you know some things, we know some things, and we'll work it out."

TEAM BUILDING

Our early training exercises (many of them designed to build a sense of group belonging in the team) often replicated experiences we had had in counseling training. They came from ideas based on modernist ideas of "getting in touch with the essential self." One evening session required each person to speak about a life experience or experiences that were significant. The group quickly became captivated by the idea that what was talked about should be difficult and traumatic experiences. The aftermath involved no sleep as tearful young people comforted one another and continued to talk about the problems they faced in their lives. So strong was dominant talk of trauma that one fifteen-year-old apologized for having nothing difficult in his life to talk about! Our discomfort with the situation and the belief system that lies behind this sort of exercise has led us to set up different evening discussion groups. (We now initiate talk about what has brought people to the work and who stands beside them as they go ahead.) Looking back, we see this as a significant step in our learning and acknowledgment of the power in our role as facilitators. Our practice now would be to speak with the team about our uncertainty with the exercise and to discuss possible outcomes, but eight or nine years ago, we acted without consultation and changed the focus. We both identify this as the only time we can remember a sense of not "working with" the students, as the team felt that the original exercise was one of the highlights of camp.

FUTURE PLANNING AND DIRECTIONS

We tried the following activity on one of the evenings during last year's camp. We began by declaring our purpose and intentions—to look at the influence of the team in the school, its strengths and its vulnerabilities—and to look at harassment's purposes, practices, and weapons in the school at the current time. We both believe that to fully include students, our thinking must be made available to them by being spoken. We also had an intention to be guarding against the possible effects of success that might lead us all into smugness and complacency. The previous year had been an eventful one for the team with much public acknowledgment and praise after a series of conference presentations and teaching workshops. We explained that this was a form of critiquing our work.

Students played roles of harassment, and the Anti-Harassment Team formed a panel at the front of the room and were interviewed by the group (Roth and Epston, 1996). One of the team took the chair to organize the process. At the end, the whole group discussed what had emerged. We asked them to think about any ideas, new thoughts, or implications that had occurred to them. The new team members contributed in this discussion and their voices were useful in that they could bring an outsider viewpoint.

Several new ideas emerged. The idea of being "resistance fighters" against harassment and the need when you have a resistance movement to be on the lookout for new recruits. In this case, the team decided that they wanted teachers as recruits in supporting and understanding their work more. They wanted to make more of a connection with the adults in the school to create a community around the work. This led to a meeting with teachers to discuss the ideas with them.

They chose a new direction for publicity which emphasized the breadth of what the team could offer and encouraged people to seek help for dealing with problems between friends as well as for harassment issues.

Part of the new publicity was to educate more people about what to expect in mediations—the even-handedness of the mediator means that even if someone feels wronged the mediator will not take sides in the mediation. This was not something we had realized to be necessary.

TRUST

Some reflections from students on the importance of adult trust seemed an appropriate way to conclude.

"If we felt we had to do a mediation because we were told to or made to, we wouldn't be passionate about trying our ideas and developing them, and wouldn't enjoy it as much. They fully trust us, that we're doing it. They never check on us; if they ask, it's to know how we are. It's not to see if we stuffed up or something. They don't watch over us."

NOTES

1. Selwyn College is a public, coeducational secondary school of 900 students ranging from thirteen years of age to adult.

BIBLIOGRAPHY

Bird, J. (2000). *The heart's narrative: Therapy and navigating life's contradictions.* Auckland, New Zealand: Edge City Press.

Bruell, A., Gatward, E., and Salesa, L. (1999). The Anti-Harassment Team: A presentation of hope. *Narrative Therapy and Community Work: A Conference Collection.* Adelaide, Australia: Dulwich Centre Publications.

Cheshire A. and Lewis, D. (2001). *Taking the Hassle Out of School* (Second Edition). A Handbook available from Selwyn College, Auckland, New Zealand.

Lewis, D. and Cheshire, A. (1998). The work of the Anti-Harassment Team of Selwyn College. *Dulwich Centre Journal* 2 and 3: 3-32.

Morgan, A. (1995). Taking responsibility: Working with teasing and bullying in schools. *Dulwich Centre Newsletter* 2 and 3: 16-29.

Roth, S. A. and Epston, D. (1996). Developing externalizing conversations: An exercise. *Journal of Systemic Family Therapy* 15(1): 5-12.

Winslade, J. and Monk, G. (1999). *Narrative Counseling in Schools.* Thousand Oaks, CA: Sage Publications.

Winslade, J. and Monk, G. (2000). *Narrative mediation: A new approach to conflict resolution.* San Francisco: Jossey-Bass.

Chapter 10

Knowing-With:
Moral Questions of Relationship

Wally McKenzie

This chapter articulates a form of *knowing-with* that has hitherto
been avoided and neglected in therapy, namely, moral questions and
decisions in relationship contexts. A moral perspective in therapy is illustrated with reference to separating couples and families, particularly in relation to the legal and court issues that accompany the termination of the family unit. McKenzie provides detailed examples of
questions that elicit moral narratives in the past and future life of the
family. These moral stories may concern lifestyle, parenting, and the
welfare of children, and are generally reflective of wider cultural discourses.

Three counseling vignettes illustrate the significance of moral stories and dilemmas in the personal lives and relationships of clients.
Such moral practices are relevant to any collaborative approach to
therapy.

I have met many couples at the termination of their family as a unit
through separation and it is usual that some legal processes become
involved. These might be legal advice, lawyers supporting each client, family court involvement, or the setting of minimum "child
maintenance payments" by the noncustodial parent. Whatever is involved, distress seems almost certain to some or all of the family
members when a legal settlement is reached without attending to the
moral dimension of relationships. This is where the importance of
moral questioning in counseling, the division of what some would
describe as, "the letter of the law or the spirit of the law," came into
focus for me. Our Western cultures have a history of validating relationships in which legalities are attended to, such as marriage, separation, dissolution, and so on as though that action in itself dealt with

the moral aspects or the moral aspects would take care of themselves once the legal process was done (Gergen and Gergen, 1983).

Drawing on a postmodern, social construction perspective, I understand there are multiple moral discourses available in a culture at any time. These multiple discourses relate to most aspects of our lives. The moral discourse I am considering here is not that of the keeping of laws or rules, the letter of the law, or the morals of law. Rather it is the set of social/personal obligations of right and wrong, of shoulds and oughts, of ethics, of personal imperatives that are particular to a person in the changing moments of his or her life. In this context moral questions would have to do with decisions a person makes about what is right and wrong and the possible (moral) outcomes that spring from these decisions, of decisions about relationships, obligations, economics, and responsibilities.

These questions are not for the display of the moral position we as counselors occupy, for we are not charged with being the moral arbiter for our clients and community. Our place is to make visible and open for question the acquired moral stance that at once holds and guides our clients so that they are more active (rather than passive) in the development of their own lives and relationships. Relationships with self and others are less likely to be misshapen and held to ransom if people are able to explore them more critically. The moral positions we each occupy today are likely to be the cultural leftovers of yesterday, passed on to us by various and mostly invisible social/cultural histories as immutable facts (Randall, 1995). This produces a cultural blindness to practiced morals that are reinforced by particularized evidence and untouched and unaffected by a myriad of contradictions. Morals are the foundation from which much of our lives are directed and should not become one of those avoided domains in counseling. Our part in this collaborative effort is to bring our ability to question with curiosity, interest, and respect as coresearchers with our clients.

In working with couples and families at the termination of their family unit, we may discuss the ways moral decisions are made for them and how they would prefer them to be made. Some questions to generate discussion include the following:

- What do you think were the moral aspects of your family life that guided your family when you were all working together as a family unit? What aspects of life did they cover? How did you come to consider certain ways of being as more appropriate for your family than others?

- Were these moral perspectives yours, your spouse's, or were they developed together for your family? In hindsight, when it came to family life, who might have provided which ideas for the guidance of your family's moral decisions?
- Do you think these moral perspectives added something important to your family life and the development of your children? Were they adopted directly from legal principles or were they based on what you and your partner believed would be good for your family? Were they different than "keeping the law"?
- The law seems to have quite an influence in the setting up of a family and in its dissolution. Do you think that you want to let the law settle the end of your hopes and dreams for your family or should we also attend to the moral aspects involved?
- What do you suppose some of those important moral aspects might be?
- What should we do if some of these moral aspects become difficult and cause contention? Do you want to ignore them for the court to decide or press on for the sort of moral outcome that you and your family would prefer?

We might get to consider such things as the future well-being of the children in terms of the lifestyle that will benefit them the most. We might get to consider the future well-being of the children in terms of the continued parenting or new parenting that will benefit them the most and the consideration of space for the practices of ensuring their emotional, physical, spiritual, and medical safety. We might also consider the differences between good mothering and good fathering and the implications of such moral ideas. We might get to consider who will look after the children when they take sick and both separated parents are working. We will likely attend to father-child connections if the children live with their mother (Epston and McKenzie at <http://www.narrativeapproaches.com/narrative% 20papers%20folders/open-heart.htm>). Also, it is likely to be very important to consider how each parent will *actively* safeguard the practices of motherhood/fatherhood of the other parent, especially when new adult partnerships are formed. We might need to consider how the children are protected from the possible acrimony that often comes between parents with separation and how they will receive encouragement for developing an appropriate relationship with the other parent.

These are questions which create a conversation that, in my experience, people enter into with interest. The purpose of such moral questioning is not to impose or insist on some better way; rather, it is to expose the taken-for-granted assumptions on which our society continues. To evaluate them as assumptions, not as a matter of *truth,* and to make space for a wider range of moral possibilities to be considered in the ongoing development of people's lives.

There are many questions we ask in the moment of counseling together with people we meet. These questions often have to do with another person's thoughts, feelings, and sometimes aspects of relationship with others, to mention a few. It seems possible that for many counselors in their training and practice, deliberate consideration is not usually given to the inclusion of what we might call moral questions—questions about how it is that a person arrives at decisions about what is or is not appropriate or "good" for them. In fact I suspect that the very idea of moral questions in psychotherapy is generally avoided, though some more recent models (such as postmodern) would not consider them out of place. The site of moral questions is most likely to be where power, gender, racism, sexual orientation, ageism, and so on exist or might exist, and these will be found in the relational context with others and self. I am proposing that unless a moral perspective is taken into our counseling work there is a good chance that the cultural base on which people rest their lives will remain untested, taken for granted, and therefore will remain in full effect. I would prefer that people were able to hold such moral perspectives up for examination before adopting them as their own (Burr, 1995).

The following vignettes are all composites from the experiences of different people I have met with in the course of my work.

FIRST VIGNETTE

It was maybe our fourth conversation together—Joan, Bob, and myself. Part way through our conversation, Joan expressed concern at the alcohol consumption of their sons and their friends on occasions in a game room at the rear of the garage. There were a number of aspects of her concern, which ranged from the volume of alcohol to the vomiting in the garden and most of all to the times when their sons and friends would run out of the game room, jump into their cars, and race down the road. On those occasions especially, Joan's heart would be in her mouth, and in her mind she would be praying that they would not have an accident and hurt someone else or themselves. Bob commented that although he did not like it, what he did not actually know about was not his business and he therefore could not do anything about it. There was a significant difference between the positions of the two parents. As a concerned mother Joan felt marginalized in her concerns, that they were not taken seriously and talked about. Whenever she spoke to her son she was abused by him and told to mind her own business and to leave him alone. Bob chose to take no (apparent) position around this, as he believed that Joan's "interference" already added fuel to the fire, that "boys will be boys," and "I remember being a young guy once and doing stupid things." Joan subsequently felt more isolated as a person, as a caring, loving mother, and she felt more distant from Bob.

It seemed that there were at least important questions of power and gender, emerging manhood, motherhood, and older/wiser manhood that could be asked (or ignored with some effect) in this situation. There were numerous possibilities, and I began to explore them.

"It seems that there could be a moral dilemma here, and I would like to ask you both about this so that I better understand the situation. I now know that you both are differently concerned about the amount of alcohol consumed, but if one night your son and his friends had been drinking and then raced off down the road in their cars and had an accident, hurting someone, how would you feel morally about the hurt inflicted on that innocent person by your alcohol-influenced son? What effect would it have on your moral conscience that you didn't actually know how much they had been drinking but that you had a strong suspicion it was too much?" Joan quickly affirmed that she thought about the possibility of an accident a lot and never wanted that on her conscience. It would be her worst nightmare. Bob, after a considerable and thoughtful pause, said, "Putting it that way I would have to say it would be absolutely terrible. I would feel like Joan."

I continued, "So considering this moral question and its possible implications for the two of you as parents, as well as your son and the wider community, what call does that make on you as a parental couple?"

Bob responded quickly with, "We have to decide together to do something about this!" The outcome was a drawing together of the two in parenting. However, from previous conversations it seemed likely to me that there was still the possibility of another moral dilemma which could easily be overlooked, that within the relationship between Joan and Bob. This was that Bob would take his own stand with their son, one which in the past had not worked very well, and leave Joan without a mother/woman/wife voice. I pursued this line of thought.

"Bob, does this statement of yours mean that you think it is important to find a solution that is satisfactory to you both as parents?"

"Yes, it must be."

"Do you have some idea about how you might do this and about how you would know that the solution was satisfactory to Joan?"

There were still other moral aspects of our conversation available to us; for example, it was possible that Bob's moral relationship with himself was violated by the earlier stance of, "what I don't see, I don't know about." Addressing such moral questions allowed both to shift from a defensive stance to working together effectively with the moral position of each being valued as the base on which they began to rebuild.

What we face together in our conversations are different moral stories competing unequally in a cultural setting for acceptance—stories of "rightness," perhaps, or of "knowing how to do what needs to be done," or some other good-intentioned reason. Nevertheless, knowing that not all stories are equal and that some carry more weight than others in our Western culture, I believe that I must be intentional about what I notice, what I ignore, and what I ask about. If not, I collude with and participate in the taken-for-granted, normalizing, moral discourses of my culture. Like Bob, I have a moral position to take (which is not the same as moralizing), and cannot say that because I do not know the details of what is happening it is of no concern in counseling.

SECOND VIGNETTE

Martha, who is now in her forties, came to counseling with a long history of being overtaken (by her own account) by alcohol and shoplifting when stressed, which was very often. She had grown up living with her mother, who was a single parent, and often witnessed the stress of her mother when she opened the mail looking for a child-support check from her absent (separated) husband and often found none. The dire lack of money at home for her mother also meant none for Martha to spend as a child, which led to her stealing quite regularly to gain friendships at school and drinking alcohol from the age of nine years. From that time on, these two things have remained a feature of Martha's life, with shoplifting incidents several times a week giving her more a sense of comfort and achievement than of having taken anything that did not belong to her. In addition, these things were having significant effects on her family of three young children and possibly threatened their future. When we talked it seemed to Martha that she had always been that way and so her activities had become "normal." She thought that her mother probably focused on survival and never stopped to think about teaching her daughter morals that would equip her for living in the community.

These are the sort of questions a moral therapist might ask Martha:

- When we review your upbringing, accepting the limited resources your mother had in those days as a single parent, what morals do you think she passed on to you as a child, girl, and young woman, that were available for you into your maturity? What might you think about the ones around alcohol and stealing?
- Is it possible when you were a child that you were inadvertently taught to be a different moral person than society now expects of you?
- If the moral person you are is different from the moral stance of the society you live in and are a part of, what do you think the implications could be for you as a person?
- Remembering your mother as you do, what moralities do you think she would have wanted for you had she not been so encumbered with the daily survival of you both while you were growing up?
- As you now entertain becoming a moral person of your own making, would she be surprised at your endeavor, your humanity, your hopes for yourself as a person, your attention to the family name, and your attention to your own place in the community?

THIRD VIGNETTE

Not long ago, I met with Sara and her son Daniel. I had been meeting with Sara for some time with regard to a number of things, including the abusive and emotionally violent nature of the relationship between she and her husband Roger and his abusive and emotionally violent relationship with their son. These outbursts were unpredictable, intimidating, and would often reduce his wife and adult son to tears, leaving them feeling worthless, devastated, and hating his company. They reported that they never felt good enough for him and could never satisfy his expectations. I remember asking Sara and Daniel, "Could you tell me whether Roger is like this in any way at all when he is at work?"

They chorused a reply, "No, at work he is a manager with about ten staff and they all love him!"

"Tell me about this. It might help me to understand things better."

Over the next ten minutes I learned that as a manager in his workplace he was well respected by the staff who worked under his management and who spoke of the ways he would take a stand for them and listen well to them. "Well," I asked, "what do you suppose his interactions with them must be like for him to be thought of in such a way? Do they receive from him what you receive?"

"No," they again chorused. "We have heard the way they talk about him."

"In that case, does it seem just a little strange that the people who don't love him and he doesn't love either get better treatment than you as the people who do love him and who he says he loves?"

Sara and Daniel realized that they had accepted the resulting relationship as uncomfortably "normal." The two explored ways of asking Roger about how it was that this situation could possibly be, ways of telling him that it was no longer acceptable for them as a family and that they would support him in changing their relationship with him to a more loving one, then left for home. Some time later I was fortunate enough to meet with Roger and Sara to talk together and make some meaning from what was happening. Roger was clear that he never had any intention of being this way with his family and affirmed that he really did love them all. His family began to take a stand against the abuse and the self-blame it invited them to invoke on themselves. Roger was invited to consider the sort of moral relationship he wanted to have with his family.

These are moral questions of the sort not previously thought through before by any of the family that a therapist might ask of Roger.

- What do you think your family would possibly make of your love for them if they take into account the outbursts that so often mark the relationship between you and them?
- When you think about it, what do you make of your love for them when you take those outbursts into account? Do they leave your love relationship with them fractured a little?
- How would you describe the love relationship these outbursts imply that you have with them?
- Would Sara and Daniel describe your relationship with them as a love relationship, a love relationship mixed with fear, or something else?
- How do the "outbursts" fit with the love relationship you want your family to experience with you? Do they reduce the effectiveness of your love for your family? What place do the outbursts have in maximizing the love for your family? When did you become aware of the limitations the "outbursts" impose in drawing your family to you?
- Are the outbursts your own invention or did you acquire them somewhere in your life?
- When you first got together with Sara did you imagine that "outbursts" would have a place in the development of your relationship with her and the family the two of you would create?
- In what ways do you think the "outbursts" limit your family's appreciation of you? How would you rather be appreciated by them?
- In what ways have the "outbursts" limited the husbanding and fathering in your family?

We thus participate in the construction of a moral identity.

FINAL THOUGHTS

The usual discourses of counseling, as socially and personally constructed, invite me into a moralizing stance with my clients—particularly as issues become overwhelmingly socially unacceptable in their effects. Therefore, I must ask moral questions of myself in my practice. These moral questions are not another "model" of counseling. They have emerged out of the postmodern, narrative practice that is my preferred way of working. They can be situated in many other paradigms if they are thought to be important by the practitioner.

- Where and how do I stand with this concern?
- What has informed this position/stand I take?
- What is my personal stand?
- Where do I want my stand to figure in this conversation?
- Where in my conversations with clients does the "truth" of my personal moral position begin to show itself as maybe a more convincing position for them?
- What is there about my client's responses in the conversation that lead me to establish the moral truth?
- What is the moral truth I might be drawn into establishing?
- How did this moral truth become a moral truth (i.e., its origin)?
- How might I make the moral aspect of my conversation "contestable" for my clients?
- What is my responsibility and its place in the context of co-research? (Epston and McKenzie, 1999)

REFERENCES

Burr, V. (1995). *An Introduction to Social Constructionism.* London: Routledge.
Epston, D. and McKenzie, W. (1999). M. Counseling degree assignment: University of Waikato, New Zealand.
Gergen, K. and Gergen, M. (1983). Narratives of the self. In Theodore, R. and Scheibe, K. (Eds.), *Studies in Social Identity.* New York: Praeger Publishers.
Randall, W. (1995). *The Stories We Are: An Essay on Self Creation.* Toronto, Canada: University of Toronto Press.

SUGGESTED READINGS

Bird, J. (1999). *The Heart's Narrative.* Auckland, New Zealand: Edge Press.
Doherty, W. J. (1995). *Soul Searching.* New York: Basic Books.
Young, I.M. (1997). *Intersecting Voices.* Princeton, NJ: Princeton University Press.

SUPERVISION AND TRAINING:
RELATIONAL PRACTICES

Chapter 11

Countercultural Therapy: An Attempt to Match Pedagogy to Practice

Kevin Fitzsimmons
Larry Zucker

> The issue of the legitimation of knowledges has been a central preoccupation of postmodernism and poses some intriguing challenges for those aspiring to "train" therapists in collaborative approaches. To adopt a primarily didactic posture and convey theory and practice is to locate expertise mostly in the domain of the instructor. It fails to capture what family therapist Karl Tomm calls a "bring-forthist" spirit—an orientation more intent on invoking than transmitting knowledge. A second concern, one voiced by many of the contributors to this book, is to avoid replacing a modern dogma with a postmodern one.
>
> Kevin Fitzsimmons and Larry Zucker are keenly focused on these issues in their work with clinicians in training. They encourage their students to adopt a countercultural posture of critical reflection toward the myriad taken-for-granted ideas and practices of psychology. In the foundational phase of their training, which they describe here, they use discussions of key readings and experiential exercises to help clinicians see beyond the surface, to pay attention to how ideas—both modern and postmodern—play out in practice.

She is nineteen, articulate, and intense. She describes ritually and regularly penetrating the skin of her forearm with a razor-sharp blade as a pleasure, a bloody relief from the pain she locates in her mind. As she speaks to the therapist she has only just met, she thinks he is listening, as therapists do, with ears sensitive to her pain and perceptive to her pathology. When she rolls up the sleeve of her sweater to reveal a map of scars on her brown skin, she believes it reveals the evidence

145

of a disturbed self. She has no way of knowing he might perceive the scars as evidence of a response that makes sense in the world in which the cutting occurred. Whether or not this world will be part of their thinking and talking will, in large part, depend on the conversational options the therapist sees as available. Will this young person's status as a female, as the daughter of immigrant parents, as a member of a racial minority, as a member of the lower-middle economic class find a relationship to her scarred skin? Or will the scars remain as they exist in the minds of her family, friends, and, as they exist in the majority of the literature meant to guide the practice of psychotherapy, as manifestations of an ill individual whose behavior is self-destructive and irrational.

Much of what the therapist in this scenario considers as she or he listens will be the result of how she or he has been taught and trained. Much of that training will characterize this young woman as having an individual illness. In our work as educators, we try to open the possibility for therapists to see and hear much that stands outside of dominant stories that the institution of therapy and the wider culture tell about clients, and the stories that clients tell about themselves. In other words, we would hope that the therapists we have influenced act with the understanding that psychotherapy involves itself in issues of power and politics. Paradoxically, we achieve this by exerting our power and our influence over the student therapists we teach and train. We have no intention of dominating them or subjugating them, and we take measures to ensure that our classes are as democratic in spirit as possible. But as teacher/trainers we *do* make decisions about what to do and why and when to do it because we have the power and the desire to do so. This, of course, situates us in a bind. We exert power over student trainees to encourage them to refrain from exerting power over clients. We think this paradox is inescapable. In navigating it, we attempt to be accountable to the ideas about psychotherapy we believe in, and how they can exist where more popular ideas prevail. We foster this accountability by adopting practices that better ensure it and recognize that prevailing ideology is like the air that we breathe. We are often unaware of that ideology as it manifests in the holding of our power as teacher/trainers. This chapter intends to reveal our current best thinking about how to teach what we teach.

We hope two themes will stand out in the writing that follows. First, we do not believe in teaching methodology. We think such teaching encourages imitation rather than connection to the assumptions that inform a distinct way of practicing. Second, and growing out of the first, we believe in teaching psychotherapy as a *countercultural* practice. By this we do not mean avant garde, but we do mean adversarial. To train a countercultural therapist is to train a therapist who understands that his or her clients are trying to rewrite their experience in a world where certain meanings are more popular than others, and who also understands that therapists—like it or not—are empowered by their culture to continue to popularize prevailing ideas regarding what is considered the best or most healthy way to be a person, be in a relationship, move through a stage of life, and so on. The kind of psychotherapy we are interested in teaching toward is a psychotherapy that counters the assumption that a therapist should be so empowered.

Our course meets weekly for eight months. It is independent of any university or college program and is affiliated with a community-based counseling center in central Los Angeles. Because of its independence, it is not required to provide its services according to funder guidelines. The students that choose to attend our courses have master's degrees in psychology or social work. Class meets for one and one half hours each week and is followed by a three-hour supervision. For the purposes of this writing, we will confine ourselves to describing the first few weeks of the class meetings, which prepare students for engaging in more specific therapeutic practices in the remainder of the course.

A pedagogy often teaches as much, if not more, than the subject matter it intends to impart. For instance, if the format for teaching is the didactic lecture mode, it teaches not only the material delivered in the lectures but also that the students lack knowledge which the lecturer possesses and is, therefore, delivering. In the case of teaching the material of postmodern approaches to psychotherapy, the flattening of the hierarchy between therapist and client is a fundamental emphasis. Consistency between material and mode, then, requires a teaching pedagogy that parallels this emphasis. For this reason, we believe that the teaching of postmodern psychotherapy should closely mirror the principles of practice. Since postmodern psychotherapy focuses on conversations that emerge from invitations to make or revise meanings, our teaching serves as an invitation into such conversation; since postmodern psychotherapy encourages countering the traditional hierarchical practices in the psychotherapy field, our teaching practices encourage countering the traditional hierarchical practices of postgraduate education; since postmodern psychotherapy promotes the expertise and established knowledges of clients, our teaching promotes the expertise and established knowledges of our students. We take the responsibility for promoting a learning context in which discovering is valued over replicating, in which bringing forth takes precedence over dictating to, and in which wondering is preferred to knowing.

In our first meeting with our students, we host a conversation regarding their individual original intentions in entering the general field of psychotherapy. We then invite them to tell the story of what has happened to these intentions since entering the field. This often elicits anecdotes of episodes in which teachers, supervisors, and colleagues have criticized, pathologized, rendered invisible, or otherwise denigrated these intentions by imposing particular theoretical "truths" on students' experiences. We perceive this kind of imposition as a form of violence, however well intended. We also hear accounts of sincerely caring authorities who, though tuned to dialogue and relationship, insist on allegiance to the supremacy of certain ideas about human nature and functioning. Although a "kinder and gentler" approach, we consider this insistence as a kind of violence as well.

Although we understand our use of the word violence might be considered extreme to some, we believe it is an accurate description of processes that often happen in the education of a psychotherapist. We also believe these processes mirror what often happens in psychotherapy. Psychotherapists are taught, trained, and supervised by experts to be experts. Generally speaking, the expertise transmitted concerns ideas considered as truths about human nature, about human functioning, and this transmission of so-called truth has profound effects on the unfolding of psychotherapy. For instance, the young woman in the opening vignette is likely to emerge from different therapists' offices with widely differing accounts of her own experience. In the office of a therapist who takes for truth the notion that cutting is "self-destructive," or focuses inquiry around "impulsivity" as an actual trait or part of her makeup, those meanings are either going to be taken as truth by the client, or they will invite a resistance that itself can then be storied as self-destructive or impulsive. Stories that might have been elicited by those who hold other truths or, better, who are wary of the truth, are thus less likely to emerge; for example, stories that might consider her cutting to be an act that preserves her integrity in the context of ongoing abuse, or cutting as a manifestation of a cultural invitation to find her current body in need of alteration.

We think of the prevailing "truths" as expressions of a mainstream therapy culture, parts of narratives that have come to be taken for granted as fundamentally and universally true. They have been taken for granted because of the authority with which they have been delivered and held. Consequently we think of them as acts of power. They serve to oppress other ideas that should be freely accessible to all who make meaning of their experiences. To authoritatively abuse another's ability to access such ideas is to do violence.

Having elicited student stories of such violence, we explore their responses to them with an ear for stories about how they have hung on to some of their original intentions. Here, students often speak of hopes and dreams that they still want to make part of their practice of psychotherapy. We wonder with them about how they have been able to hang on to these intentions while journeying through territory where such intentions are either not seen or seen and not allowed. We understand their ability to keep certain intentions, hopes, and dreams alive as evidence of their resistance to violence. Together, we explore ways we can work together that will not duplicate the relational violence they have experienced in the field. So prepared, we embark on an exploration of literature that reflects on the socially constructed foundations of meaning—including the meaning of the readings themselves.

In introducing our first reading, we emphasize that we offer all of our readings and exercises as invitations to think critically about the foundational truths of contemporary psychotherapy. Although our hope is to establish the socially constructed nature of these foundations, it is not to incite an oppositional tension toward these ideas disguised as truth but to incite a reaction to the use of authority involved in the disguise itself. Our intention is not to promote debate between people with differing beliefs. Rather, it is to validate responses that question the elevation of belief to Truth, and that question the authority of those people and processes which do the elevating.

Over time, the readings we select continue to evolve in response to students' input. What makes them noteworthy is that they are not devoted to explaining client experience or techniques for altering that experience. Instead, we focus on the study of a psychotherapist's *relationship* to knowledge and on the effect that relationship to knowledge has on the lives of our clients. As holders of master's degrees in psychology or social work, our students are amply steeped in the gathered knowledge of the profession, and we do not see our role as transmitters of even more. Thus we frequently witness students developing practices not out of these knowledges but from beliefs and values that emerge from our mutual exploration. In this sense, method is not conveyed, but emerges in much the same way as client knowledges emerge in postmodern collaborative therapy.

Before proceeding with these challenging readings, we believe it best to establish a position of respect toward the dignities of modernist thought. In our most recent class we did this by providing Chapter 1 of Ken Wilber's (1998) *The Marriage of Sense and Soul.* Situating modernist thought, Western civilization, and scientific enlightenment historically, he highlights the dignified intentions of using knowledge to reduce human suffering, to foster equality, and to promote individual liberty. Simultaneously, he exposes the disasters associated with modernism, the overarching one being a scientism that robs experience of its authority in making meaning and concurrently dissipates curiosity about mysteries not yet understood.

With this established, we promote discussion about dignified and disastrous aspects of the contemporary education of a psychotherapist, again with an ear for stories of resistance to the disastrous side of that experience. Our first experiential exercise imbeds these ideas in a written, contemporary mental health evaluation of a boy depicted as "severely emotionally disturbed" and in need of psychotherapeutic services. Collectively, we examine not the content but the writing style of the piece as if doing a literary analysis. Literary devices are brought forth from this analysis, such as the choice of the writer to use the third-person omniscient point of view, to consistently favor passive voice constructions, to prefer intransitive verbs over those of action, and so on. We then confirm that for the majority of us this is a recognizable and familiar style common to documents produced in the mental health professions, the "taken-for-granted" way of using language and a way of transmitting authority for the professionals in the mental health field. Noticing this allows us to reflect on how easy it is to use language in taken-for-granted ways without being accountable to its effect. For instance, to casually use the taken-for-granted term "self-destructive" in describing the young woman in our vignette is to profoundly shape her biography, yet many would do so without hesitation. Some even use report-writing software that has such assumptive truth built into its database of boilerplate descriptions. Here, we begin to encourage an honest speculation about what it requires of a person who does not agree with taken-for-granted ideas about authority to use language consciously in a profession that prefers that she or he did not. This discussion brings us back to the theme of dignities and disasters, and to the awareness of how the preferred use of language reflects and reinforces social constructions of reality.

The second reading we review is a chapter from Robert Fancher's (1995) *Cultures of Healing.* This chapter, "Care As Culture," articulately explores the world of mental health and sensitively establishes that, at its best, it is a field of the best guess when it comes to relieving human suffering. The concept of culture illuminates how beliefs and practices not necessitated by nature are deemed to be natural truths. Fancher compassionately avoids humiliating the practitioners and practices of such a culture by arguing for the dignity of the impulse to do the best one can to alleviate human suffering. He does, however, question the inability of the field to note its own culture-bound truth claims. The discussion naturally finds its way back to points about the use of language as one of the ways a culture of healing attempts to maintain its claims to authoritative truth. The question it prompts is how one can practice without adherence to the truth claims of "cultures of care" and with full recognition of the culture-bound nature of its ideas.

Though experiential exercises follow each reading, space limits us to summary description here. The following question hovers throughout our Fancher-related experiential exercise:

> If the knowing of schools of psychotherapy is in large part cultural, subjective, and not scientific, and if the expertise/knowledge claims can be viewed as acts of persuasion, how might we practice in ways that hold ourselves accountable for the persuasive effects—intended or not—of our own acts?

In a role-play exercise, a consultant who is authorized to "interrupt" or "start over" a therapy session helps a therapist stay interested in the aforementioned question while experimenting with various questions, intentionalities, and interviewing practices. The exercise reveals some of the specific challenges in preferring a therapy intent on accounting for the biases of cultures of care. For example, recent students have struggled with questions of separating oppressive pseudo-science from useful science, finding a balance between abusing authority and having no influence on what transpires in a session, and declining certainty about human nature at the risk of appearing inexperienced to their clients. These then are posed to be some of the challenges the course must face if it is to be truly useful to the development of congruent practices.

The next reading, "Selves, Illnesses, Healers, and Technologies," is a chapter from *Constructing the Self, Constructing America,* in which the historian/therapist author, Phillip Cushman (1995), suggests that concepts central to the practices of psychotherapy are reflections of the sociopolitical historical context during which they flourish. Cushman emphasizes that what is cultural is socially constructed. This is true about ideas of what the self is; in other words, the self is not a universal, transhistorical concept. Consequently, illnesses of the self are culture- and era-bound, as are the treatments meant to address them. By this point in the course, discrepancies between prevailing cultural values and the values held by individual students have become a significant focus of discussion. The conversation begins to elicit student thoughts regarding integrity of practice, building on ideas of previous class discussions as it centers on the commitment to developing knowledge, material, and methodology congruent with values.

Cushman's chapter is prefaced by a quote from a Kurt Vonnegut (1971) novel concerning the planet of Tralfamadore, where, among other differences, meaning is not made in a linear fashion. Our reading of Cushman is followed by an exercise like the last, where therapist, client, and consultant—in this case a Tralfamadorian—work together to make more visible the weaving of culture-bound assumption into the moment-by-moment practice of psychotherapy. For example, a Tralfamadorian consulting to the therapist in our opening vignette might wonder why someone who still existed was being referred to as self-destructive. On Tralfamadore people exist only as long as they will it.

Our fourth reading is a chapter by Joel Pfister (1997) in a book of essays he edited with Nancy Schnog called *Inventing the Psychological* (Pfister and Schnog, 1997). The chapter, "On Conceptualizing the Cultural History of Emotional and Psychological Life in America," agrees with Cushman's notion that what is considered psychological in our culture is an expression of the culture. Pfister, after focusing on how psychological language presents human nature as understood and therefore potentially under control, foreshadows his contextualizing the "inventing of the psychological" within the cultural history of power. As he does so, he is able to point out psychology's complicity with the maintenance of racist, classist, sexist, and homophobic ideas in America. The discussion of this chapter gives all a chance to muse about the issue of power as related to psychotherapy, about the taken-for-granted nature of that power, of the irony of the "helping" profession's penchant for claiming it lives outside the realms of power and therefore politics. When all is said and done, the chapter serves to bring forth the idea that psychotherapy is political.

The ensuing exercise begins with the students reading a pseudo-client letter written to his new psychotherapist. It details the problems he is experiencing and the background he finds pertinent to include. He describes the ending of a relationship, difficulties with feelings of sadness, anger, loss of normal interest in the opposite sex, difficulty sleeping, and feelings of failure related to this and other relationships ending. He puts the relationship in a cultural context by describing himself and his ex-fiancé as having different class and racial backgrounds. He mentions his strong mother, the two sisters he is flanked by and close to, and his long-absent father. He mentions the possibility that his father may have had manic-depressive illness and/or misused alcohol. The exercise calls for the students to assume they are the therapist and to reflect on the letter in three ways. First they are to list all the popular ideas of contemporary psychology the letter brings to their minds. Then they are asked to list what they glean are the client's rationale and assumptions in seeking therapy, based on his own words and meanings as they understand them. Finally, they are asked to list the contexts and discourses of contemporary culture—including the discourses of therapy itself—not necessarily directly spoken of that the letter brings forth for them.

The first category of prevailing ideas in the current cultures of psychotherapy contains ideas familiar to anyone familiar with popular psychology in Western culture. Ideas in this first category may be individualistic ("low self-esteem") or systemic ("middle child"); pathologizing ("controlling mother, absent father") or normalizing ("stage of grief"); professional ("developmental fixation") or pop ("mid-life crisis,"); biological ("chemical imbalance") or social ("fear of commitment"). The items in this category have several commonalities: they are all explanatory rather than descriptive, they all exist as valid explanations with strong preexisting constituencies; and they all leap readily to our minds and, likely, to our clients' minds.

The second category, frequently and unfortunately squeezed by traditional training into the client's "chief complaint," begins as a simple list of things the client has most directly addressed as his concerns: feeling "abnormal" in his lack of desire, worrying about the accruing effects of disturbed sleep, feeling like a "failure" in relationship, concerned about the possibility of "depression" as he understands it.

The third category concerns discourse, less familiar to therapists though more recognized by sociologists, cultural anthropologists, or linguists. It concerns the larger frames of reference within which meaning making unfolds. In the case example, students might examine discourse concerning mental health and who is empowered to define it, substance use and misuse and who is empowered to distinguish one from the other, race as a concept that has culturally shifting meanings, class as an invisible issue that is affecting how therapist, client, and his ex-partner might feel differently entitled in relation to each other, unmarried status as a suspect state, gendered ideas about relationship and who is responsible for creating and maintaining it, and "self " as taken-for-granted locus of feelings and experience.

These three categories (popular psychological explanation, client's stated experience and wishes, and prevailing discourse) we regard as the contents of a countercultural therapist's consciousness. This exercise has tended to produce a "three category" metaphor that organizes much of the rest of the course, and it is used to make sense of student as well as client experience. The first and third categories reflect cultural constructions, ways of making sense that might either illuminate or obscure lived experience. The middle category of initially presented description is treated as a starting point for conversation, and the purpose of ensuing conversation is to stretch or widen this category so that the evolving descriptions come ever-closer to matching actual lived and living experience, and have increasingly freeing effects. For instance, the young woman in our opening vignette might prefer the effects of understanding her history of cutting to be self-preserving rather than self-destroying, or a student in the course may prefer to think of her or his intent to help as coming from her or his dream of a preferred world rather than, for instance, a result of being a middle child. In general, we believe that what emerges is a richer description of lived experience, made richer by a therapy that listens for how life's meanings can be distorted by devotion to prevailing ideas in the field and can be enhanced by situating these meanings in the culture at large.

The learning experiences we have been describing here are the foundation that we build with students in preparation for the development of their unique therapeutic methods. Our task through this process is to consistently support students' efforts to develop practices that meet the challenges prompted by their initially stated intentions and by the readings, discussions, and exercises that have followed. This support takes the form of encouraging a careful use of language, a careful attention to client resources, and a careful allegiance to client preferences. In supervision we restrain the corrective impulse supported by our years of experience in favor of questions that promote further reflection. We have witnessed such questioning and reflection incite students toward the development of practices that adhere to foundational assumptions. This commitment is distinct from the commitment to replicate the practices of another whose ideas are admired; rather, it is a commitment to one's own capacity to transform assumption into action. What often emerges is methodology resulting more firmly from belief than imitation. It is our intention to use our teaching opportunity to bring forth a student's commitments. We find this encouragement of a reflexive and intentional disposition is not only beneficial to students and their current and future clients but also fits with our commitments as teachers.

REFERENCES

Cushman, P. (1995). *Constructing the Self, Constructing America: A Cultural History of Psychotherapy*. Reading, MA: Addison-Wesley Publishing Company.

Fancher, R. (1995). *Cultures of Healing: Correcting the Image of American Mental Health Care*. New York: W. H. Freeman and Company.

Pfister, J. and Schnog, N. (1997). *Inventing the Psychological: Toward a Cultural History of Emotional Life in America.* New Haven, CT: Yale University Press.

Vonnegut, K. (1971). *Slaughterhouse Five: Or Children's Crusade, A Duty-Dance with Death.* New York: Dell Publishing.

Wilber, Ken. (1998). *The Marriage of Sense and Soul: Integrating Science and Religion.* New York: Random House.

SUGGESTED READINGS

The spirit with which this list is best understood is that these were readings our students found particularly helpful in figuring out their beliefs, stances, and methods as therapists in training. These readings were neither assigned nor read in the spirit of "this is how to do it"; rather, they were read for their inspiration value regarding where to stand in relation to clients' difficulties.

Freeman, J., Epson, D., and Lobovits, D. (1997). *Playful Approaches to Serious Problems: Narrative Therapy with Children and Their Families.* New York: W. W. Norton (Particularly Chapter 10, "Weird and Special Abilities," pp. 179-192).

Jenkins, A. (1990). *Invitations to Responsibility: The Therapeutic Engagement of Men Who Are Violent and Abusive.* Adelaide, Australia: Dulwich Centre Publications. (Particularly Part II, The Process of Engagement of Men Who Abuse Their Partners, pp. 59-100).

Wade, A. (1997). Small Acts of Living: Everyday Resistance to Violence and Other Forms of Oppression. *Contemporary Family Therapy,* 19(1) March 1977. Human Sciences Press.

White, M. (1997). *Narratives of Therapists' Lives.* Adelaide, Australia: Dulwich Centre Press (Particularly Part III: The Ethic of Collaboration and Decentered Practice).

Winslade, J. and Monk, G. (1999). *Narrative Counseling in Schools: Powerful and Brief.* Thousand Oaks, CA: Corwin Press, Inc. (Particularly Chapter 3: "Reworking Reputations").

Chapter 12

Introducing Social Constructionist and Critical Psychology into Clinical Psychology Training

David J. Harper

David Harper's chapter concerns the teaching and training of clinical psychologists; specifically, how trainees can develop knowing and expertise within a relevant reflective practice model. This does not negate but builds on a scientist-practitioner model, allowing psychology trainees to access a range of knowledge practices. Psychological knowledge can include the use of personal experience and admit uncertainty or not-knowing where required. Harper describes a training workshop and various strategies to facilitate awareness of the relationship between the personal and professional in therapist's lives. Here therapists gently deconstruct the us-and-them thinking that demarcates psychologists from service users or mental health system survivors. This provides a foundation for trainees to develop empathic knowing-with in their clinical work.

The chapter looks at how collaborative practices and ideas can be introduced into mainstream clinical psychology training. It provides examples of qualitative assessment in writing up case study reports and describes the operation of reflective practitioner groups. It concludes with a useful exercise in narrative supervision for trainees and supervisors to evaluate clinical placements.

INTRODUCTION

In this chapter I want to suggest some ways of introducing ideas from social constructionist and critical psychology into a generic, mainstream training context, specifically clinical psychology training. Given the emphasis elsewhere in this volume on theory and research, this chapter will focus on concrete and practical suggestions for trainers across a variety of domains: teaching, assessment of case study material, the development of a professional identity, and clinical placements. What is offered on training courses is obviously influenced by their contexts, which I will first briefly describe.

CONTEXTS FOR TRAINING

In the United Kingdom, clinical psychology is a three-year, full-time postgraduate doctoral training, with trainees usually being salaried employees of the National Health Service (NHS). It is a generic training in terms of client groups covered (adults, older adults, people with learning disabilities, children and adolescents, and some specialist areas); theoretical orientation (cognitive-behavioral, psychodynamic, and systemic on many courses); and areas of practice (assessment, therapeutic interventions, and research, evaluation, and consultancy). Trainees receive both academic teaching (mainly from practicing clinical psychologists) and clinical experience via placements of roughly six months.

There are a number of constraints on the training offered. Training courses must receive accreditation by the British Psychological Society and also have to meet quality and other targets made by the bodies that purchase training. In addition, courses have to meet certain academic regulations since most courses are offered through universities and so have exams and other assessed work, as well as a final research dissertation. Assessment of clinical work is conducted by placement supervisors who determine whether a trainee has passed his or her placement. As a result of these different mechanisms there is a lot of similarity between clinical psychology training courses. However, these different pressures often pull in opposite directions with, for example, academic demands being in tension with practice demands.

These contexts generate a number of dilemmas for trainers wanting to introduce ideas from critical and social constructionist psychology. One dilemma here as with other generic courses is how to introduce such ideas within a very busy teaching and clinical experience curriculum. Another is how to balance theoretical teaching alongside more practical and skills-based teaching. Yet another is how to manage the tension between encouraging critical and innovative thinking with the need to "pass" course requirements—a very tricky problem, as Crocker (1998) illustrates. A further dilemma is how to introduce complex ideas without on the one hand confusing trainees, while on the other hand avoiding becoming overly pragmatic and losing a critical edge. Courses are aiming to produce clinical psychologists prepared to work in the NHS rather than social constructionists, critical psychologists, or family therapists, and course staff are not necessarily being employed to be critical psychologists or social constructionists. Moreover, critical ideas may be taught in one session, only to be followed by a less critical session taught by somebody else. Similarly, trainees may experience critical teaching but be working on placement with relatively uncritical supervisors. As a result then, critical teaching must be tactical and flexible, and my own viewpoint is to expose trainees to critical ideas and practice with an eye toward them forming their own views on what kind of clinical psychologists they want to be. I will give some brief examples of how these ideas can be introduced into different aspects of training.

PRACTICE EXAMPLES IN ACADEMIC TEACHING

From the Scientist-Practitioner to the Critical and Reflective Practitioner

In British clinical psychology the historically dominant model for integrating theory and practice has been that of the *scientist practitioner*. There have been a number of cogent critiques of this model, not least of which is that, since the majority of clinical psychologists do not regularly publish in scientific journals and do not read them often, it is more of a rhetorical ideal than a reality (Pilgrim and Treacher, 1992). The way the "scientist" part is often formulated is to privilege certain ways of doing science, usually quantitative categorical and diagnostic methods published in mainstream psychology journals. The scientist-practitioner approach has been reinforced by the advent of the evidence-based practice movement. How can one create a context where trainees can learn to develop their practice while also enabling them to deconstruct notions of "expert knowledge"—and this at a time when they are feeling the need for some certainties and security?

In teaching on this topic at the University of East London clinical training program, I have found it helpful to outline alternatives to that of a narrowly defined scientist-practitioner. Recently, models relating theory and practice that are more consistent with critical and social constructionist approaches have emerged, including that of the reflective practitioner (Clegg, 1998; Schön, 1987; Walsh and Scaife, 1998). Clegg (1998) notes that it differs sharply from notions of technical rationality:

> Schön argues that expert practitioners can easily be identified and agreed by peers in any given situation, with consensus focusing upon personal qualities such as wisdom, integrity and intuition. Research-based knowledge is accessed during this process, but it is combined with knowledge of other cases which bear some similarity and with subjective, emotional perceptions about the particular therapeutic relationship or context. (p. 7)

Schön's reflective practitioner approach has the potential to encourage trainees to reflect on their work from a number of perspectives, for example, from thinking about the influence of personal experience to interpreting their work in accordance with theory or empirical work of relevance. This model draws on similar philosophies of learning to those described by Kolb, Rubin, and McIntyre (1974) and Andersen (1992):

practice → reflection / theorizing → practice → reflection / theorizing

Indeed, some have argued that there is a need for new forms of knowledge and enquiry, specifically not applying some abstract knowledge to practice, but rather developing practice-based knowledge, or a "knowledge of practice" (Hoshmand and Polkinghorne, 1992). Since many trainees were, in a sense, waiting to get on a training course to learn the expert secrets of how to "do" therapy and since they are exposed both to course assessment requirements and a professional culture that celebrates technical rationality, they often can be left feeling bewildered and confused. In this context it can be helpful to draw on Mason's (1993) concept of *safe uncertainty*. Given that therapy is an uncertain endeavor, there is a tendency to want to be certain. Safe certainty is when we approach therapy thinking that we know the answers to all problems. This is a viewpoint that is likely to end up with many clients feeling dissatisfied (finding their difficulties transformed by the therapist into something they feel they have the answer to) or therapists feeling overwhelmed by the responsibility of having to have a solution for everything. In embracing uncertainty we do not want clients, their therapists, or trainees to feel unsafe. Exercises in which trainees are invited to examine the effects of expert knowledge models in their professional lives can be useful here since they often are at the sharp end of the theory-practice divide, where they are taught expert solutions only to find real life more complicated (Bostock, 1990; Spellman and Harper, 1996).

This approach can be helpful in learning "not knowing" approaches to therapy that avoid premature certainty and value respectfulness and curiosity (Andersen, 1992; Anderson and Goolishian, 1992). However, as a trainee in the course on which I currently work stated, "It's hard to 'not know' when you feel you really don't know." So it is important to develop an approach that sustains a safe uncertainty. Thus, it can be useful to draw a distinction between certain kinds of knowledge and expertise that we hope trainees will gain while they are in training (e.g., about therapeutic techniques or knowledge of the possible life experiences that have led to problems) and the *use* of that knowledge in particular situations. Such an approach has much in common with Larner's (2001) *critical practitioner.*

In this respect a social constructionist approach can be helpful to trainees. As Dallos and Draper (2000) note, since social constructionism is not a theory as such but rather a metatheoretical framework (i.e., a theory about theories), a social constructionist perspective allows trainees to use other theories in a pragmatic and flexible manner rather than seeing the theories or formulations which flow from them as in some foundationalist sense "true." Thus Carr (2000) has proposed that social constructionist therapists should take empirical research into effectiveness into account but, since formulations of problems and exceptions to those problems are social constructions they should not be seen as "truths." Instead the value of a formulation of a client's difficulties and of professional interventions needs to be judged by more pragmatic criteria of whether an approach "fits" for a client or is going to be useful. Gergen has talked of the importance of the notion of "usefulness" as a criterion of what count as better theories and practices in particular contexts (Misra, 1993). General evidence needs to be weighed against the particularities of the individual case. As I have noted, the aim here is not to produce social constructionist clinical psychologists but, rather, practitioners who, regardless of orientation and client group, will work collaboratively on what consumers define as their goals with respect, openness, and flexibility. There is, of course, a danger here of fostering an overly pragmatic approach and Willig (1997) has warned that a focus only on tactics—the strategic, context-specific choices one makes based on one's principles and commitments—is misconceived since "tactics must flow from a position which itself cannot be the result of tactical choices."

Thus, it is also important to discuss the ethical and political consequences of choices the practitioner might make. For example, while therapists may be influenced by critical and social constructionist ideas, the notion of a postmodernist therapy is a bit of a misnomer since therapy is inevitably a modernist endeavor (Frosh, 1995). However, if you are going to engage in therapy there are some less harmful ways of going about it. As a result it is also important to help clients judge what is and is not useful for them.

Deconstructing Us-and-Them Thinking

One effect of expert knowledge approaches to training is that they often make a clear distinction between professionals and the people who use services. Consumers of services are often seen as Other (Thomas, 1997) and some have called this an example of us-and-them thinking. This can invite professionals to act in ways experienced by consumers as lacking in ordinary human qualities. For professionals, too, this can be a strain, and many feel a split between their professional persona and their self outside of work. One way of challenging this is to link professionals' personal lives with their practice, but not in the way that much training often does—by seeking to diagnose and pathologize professionals. Rather, there is a need for a celebration of life as it is really lived by professionals (Anderson, 1995; White, 1997; White and Hales, 1997). For example, increasing numbers of professionals are "coming out" about past and ongoing mental health problems (May, 2000).

Another way of challenging the consumer/professional opposition is through more involvement of consumers of services both in feedback about therapy and in training courses. Seeking the views of consumers should become a central aspect of therapy, rather than tagged on after. They can be seen as consultants on themselves and on the difficulties they have faced and allied with in the therapy process.

Consumers need to become centrally involved in training; otherwise how are professionals to know what is really helpful to them? Consumers, especially those active in the wider survivor movement, can be invited to teach—although it is often helpful for this not to be just a "personal experience" slot but an opportunity to make more general comments about services and professionals.

Together with my colleagues Anne Cooke and Rufus May, I have helped facilitate a daylong workshop at the Salomons South East Thames course on similar topics. One exercise involves trainees thinking together in small groups about other psychologists who they think have got the balance between being a person and a professional about right. Then they are asked to recall times when they themselves feel they have got the balance right and to consider what factors influenced this. Another exercise involves trainees interviewing one another in pairs about a change they have made in their lives; a problem they have overcome, or something from which they have recovered. They are asked to explore what things helped in this process. This can help trainees recognize that people draw on many different kinds of support, resources, and personal qualities—not just those that might be regarded as professional. Then the trainees are asked to reflect on whether there were any ways in which they could appropriately draw on this experience (i.e., not just to tell a client "this worked for me so you should do it"!).

A further exercise explores the politics of what is considered normal. In groups of three the trainees are asked to take turns briefly describing an experience that might be regarded by others as unusual, for example, seeing a ghost or a UFO. In the groups they are asked to think about not only the possible meaning and causes of these events but also how they feel in telling their fellow group members. Some found this a powerful exercise, as the myth that we as professionals are always 'rational' was undermined and the significance of social reactions to things seen as abnormal or crazy was understood.

The Use of Evidence in the Assessment of Case Study Reports

As I have already noted, clinical psychology has largely embraced the evidence-based practice movement, but often what is regarded as evidence is unnecessarily narrow. One response to this is simply to broaden the notion of what constitutes "science" and "evidence" away from simplistic modernist views (Corrie and Callahan, 2000). As Larner (2001) notes "the choice is not between psychological science and non-science, but between an exclusive logical-positivist and a critical science" (p. 40).

Such concerns can come to the fore for trainees when they write up case study course assignments in which they are asked not to simply make assertions but to support claims with evidence. Sometimes this can be viewed in an overly simplistic manner, with diagnostic, psychometric instruments being the main measure of outcome or, alternatively, with the notion of measurement being inadequately dismissed. Quantitative evidence can be particularly helpful in making comparisons over time and in succinctly conveying information. However, quantitative evidence need not be based on ratings of broad diagnostic categories or on group means, which convey little about the individual case. They can, for example, include measures that focus on individual phenomena such as "symptoms." Indeed, Besa (1994) has even used a simple, single-case design to evaluate narrative therapy. Methods such as the personal questionnaire can be used, which attempt to define problems in the client's words and concepts rather than those of the therapist (Shapiro, 1961). Given that many outcome measures are practitioner-derived, consumer-focused evaluation methods can also be used (Perkins, 2000; Rogers et al., 1997). It is important, however, to match one's approach to evidence with one's theoretical paradigm. However, numerical evidence need not be based on problem- and pathology-saturated notions such as symptoms. Ratings based on solution-focused therapy rating scales can be used to measure progress toward collaboratively-defined goals. More qualitative data can be useful, for example, by drawing on clients' responses to questions such as "what is different now at the end of therapy?" Changes in the client's relationship to various domains of power can also be mapped (Hagan and Smail, 1997a,b). Quotes from interview transcripts (rather than the trainee therapist's interpretations of his or her clients' words) can be used and analyzed using a variety of qualitative research methods (e.g., discourse analysis, Kogan and Gale, 1997). Of course, trainees can also be encouraged to write case studies as personal narratives, though such work may have to be nonassessed (Green, 1989). It is important, as Larner (2001) notes, not to set up false oppositions between theoretical paradigms.

However, it is also important to help trainees understand potential conflicts and contradictions between different orientations and paradigms and to know how to integrate ideas and methods in a (trans) theoretically consistent manner rather than an eclectic or internally inconsistent hotchpotch.

The Development of a Professional Identity

I have already discussed ways in which the notion of the reflective practitioner can be introduced in teaching, but trainees also need to think through how to follow such an approach in practical contexts and how to draw on personal issues in developing as professionals. Walsh and Scaife (1998) have discussed setting up reflective practitioner groups in which trainees are encouraged to discuss their work and think through some of these dilemmas. In developing similar groups for trainees on the University of Liverpool Clinical Psychology Training scheme with Tricia Hagan, Bev Davies, Susan Mitzman, and Richard Whitehead, we outlined some guiding principles: that although personal issues might be touched on, the groups were not intended to be therapy groups; that although experiences with clients might be discussed, these were not supervision groups; that although aspects of course teaching and organization might be discussed, these were not part of a course-feedback system; and that the groups were not part of course assessment. The groups were not facilitated by course staff but by local clinical psychologists. We suggested that trainees might be encouraged to reflect on a number of issues, some of which were influenced by ideas derived from narrative therapy practitioners. Questions included:

- What kind of clinical psychologist do I want to be?
- How does my development as both a clinical psychologist and a professional relate to me as a person?
- How can I develop in a way that enables me to move between roles as a therapist, consultant, researcher, supervisor, teacher, and so on without feeling overwhelmed and confused about my role?
- How do I make sense of powerful emotional experiences on my clinical placement (e.g., with clients, supervisors, or organizational systems)?

- How might I learn from my experiences in my year group about how groups and wider systems function?
- How might I start to develop an "internal supervisor" to help in the reflective process?

Clinical Placements and Supervision

Within an expert knowledge approach to training, supervisors are seen as having more knowledge and as teaching and evaluating the performance of trainees. Introducing critical and social constructionist ideas here can be a challenge, since supervisors work with different client populations and within different theoretical orientations. Again, the aim here is not to produce social constructionist supervisors but rather supervisors who are oriented to the needs, goals, and preferences of their supervisees—for example, their preferred learning style.

Within the narrative therapy community there have been some innovative contributions to rethinking traditional ideas about supervision. White (1992) critiques the tendency in the training of therapists toward the subjugation of trainees' knowledge and the encouragement of trainees to simply copy their supervisors. He notes that attempts to copy are often met with failure, but rather than see this as a problem to be controlled, he is interested in what is originated in the attempt to copy. In other words, what is it that trainees bring of themselves to their work? Similarly, Parry and Doan (1994) see the supervisor as "an editor, a catalyst—as one who helps 'call forth' the type of therapist the trainee wishes to be, rather than as one who defines the type of therapist she/he should be" (p. 195). White (1992) has discussed one approach to helping delineate the unique qualities of trainees. He interviews them using a reflecting team, listening for "the more sparkling facts of the interviewee's counseling career" and then helping them understand how they "connect to the ideas and practices that they found in the training course into which they had enrolled" (p. 90).

Working on the assumption that one way of helping supervisors to work in this way would be to experience this approach themselves, some supervisor training workshops at the University of Liverpool utilized a short exercise. Supervisors were split into pairs for about fifteen to twenty minutes to interview each other, asking questions such as the following:

- Who and what have been some of the important influences on your development as a supervisor?
- When you think back to people who have supervised you in the past, what would you say you found most helpful about their approaches?
- If you were to track your own history and development as a supervisor, what changes would you see in your supervisory practice over time? What led to these changes?
- How would you characterize your own supervisory practice? What models and metaphors are most influential?
- What aspects of your style have trainees commented on and said were helpful to them?
- What do you like most about your own style of supervision?
- What aspects of your style would you most like to see develop in the future?
- What forms of help (e.g., training, books, and so on) would you need to support these developments?

On clinical placements, too, these ideas can be useful. Most clinical psychology courses visit placements to meet with trainees and their supervisors to review how the placement is going. This can set up a number of dynamics, for example, with both supervisor and trainee feeling they are being evaluated. While there is an evaluation element, the midplacement review can also be a time for helping both trainee and supervisor reflect on their relationship and on the trainee's unique way of learning. It can be helpful to ask supervisors, in the presence of the trainee, about the trainee's unique qualities and skills since they often have a wealth of experience with other trainees to draw on in order to make respectful comparisons. These can help the trainee to begin to develop his or her professional identity.

REFERENCES

Andersen, T. (1992). Reflections on reflecting with families. In S. McNamee and K.J. Gergen (Eds). *Therapy As Social Construction* (pp. 54-68). London: Sage.

Anderson, H. and Goolishian, H. (1992). The client is the expert: A not-knowing approach to therapy. In S. McNamee and K.J. Gergen (Eds). *Therapy As Social Construction* (pp. 25-39). London: Sage.

Anderson, L. (Ed). (1995). *Bedtime Stories for Tired Therapists*. Adelaide, Australia: Dulwich Centre Publications.

Besa, D. (1994). Evaluating narrative family therapy using simple-system research engines. *Research on Social Work Practice* 4: 309-325.

Bostock, J. (1990). Clinical training and clinical reality. *British Psychological Society Psychotherapy Section Newsletter* 8: 2-7.

Carr, A. (2000). Family Therapy: Concepts, Process and Practice. Chichester, UK: Wiley.

Clegg, J. (1998). *Critical Issues in Clinical Practice*. London: Sage.

Corrie, S. and Callahan, M.M. (2000). A review of the scientist-practitioner model: Reflections on its potential contribution to counseling psychology within the context of current health care trends. *British Journal of Medical Psychology* 73: 413-427.

Crocker, A. (1998). Learning to fail. *Context: A Magazine for Family Therapy and Systemic Practice* 39: 10-12.

Dallos, R. and Draper, R. (2000). *An Introduction to Family Therapy: Systemic Theory and Practice*. Buckingham, England: Open University Press.

Frosh, S. (1995). Postmodernism versus psychotherapy. *Journal of Family Therapy* 17: 175-190.

Green, D. (1989). Tales of discovery: Narrative approaches to training clinical psychologists. *British Psychological Society Psychotherapy Section Newsletter* 7: 28-36.

Hagan, T. and Smail, D. (1997a). Power-mapping—I. Background and basic methodology. *Journal of Community and Applied Social Psychology* 7: 257-267.

Hagan, T. and Smail, D. (1997b). Power-mapping—II. Practical application: The example of child sexual abuse. *Journal of Community and Applied Social Psychology* 7: 269-284.

Hoshmand, L.T. and Polkinghorne, D.E. (1992). Redefining the science-practice relationship and professional training. *American Psychologist* 47: 55-66.

Kogan, S.M. and Gale, J.E. (1997). Decentering therapy: Textual analysis of a narrative therapy session. *Family Process* 36: 101-126.

Kolb, D.A., Rubin, I.M., and McIntyre, J.M. (1974). *Organizational Psychology: An Experiential Approach*. Englewood Cliffs, NJ: Prentice-Hall.

Larner, G. (2001). The critical-practitioner model in therapy. *Australian Psychologist* 36: 36-43.

Mason, B. (1993). Towards positions of safe uncertainty. *Human Systems: The Journal of Systemic Consultation and Management* 4: 189-200.

May, R. (2000). Routes to recovery from psychosis: The roots of a clinical psychologist. *Clinical Psychology Forum* 146: 6-10.

Misra, G. (1993). Psychology from a constructionist perspective: An interview with Kenneth J. Gergen. *New Ideas in Psychology* 11: 399-414.

Parry, A. and Doan, R. (1994). *Story Re-Visions: Narrative Therapy in the Post-Modern World*. New York: Guilford.

Perkins, R. (2000). Solid evidence? *OpenMind* 101(January/February): 6.

Pilgrim, D. and Treacher, A. (1992). *Clinical Psychology Observed*. London: Routledge.

Rogers, E.S., Chamberlin, J., Ellison, M.L., and Crean, T. (1997). A consumer-constructed scale to measure empowerment among users of mental health services. *Psychiatric Services* 48: 1042-1047.

Schön, D.A. (1987). *Educating the Reflective Practitioner*. San Francisco: Jossey-Bass.

Shapiro, M.B. (1961). A method of measuring psychological changes specific to the individual patient. *British Journal of Medical Psychology* 34: 151-155.

Spellman, D. and Harper, D.J. (1996). Failure, mistakes, regret and other subjugated stories in family therapy. *Journal of Family Therapy* 18: 205-214.

Thomas, P. (1997). *The Dialectics of Schizophrenia*. London: Free Association Books.

Walsh, S. and Scaife, J. (1998). Mechanisms for addressing personal and professional development in clinical training. *Clinical Psychology Forum* 115: 21-24.

White, C. and Hales, J. (Eds.) (1997). *The Personal Is the Professional: Therapists Reflect on Their Families, Lives and Work*. Adelaide, Australia: Dulwich Centre Publications.

White, M. (1992). Family therapy training and supervision in a world of experience and narrative. In D. Epston and M. White (Eds.), *Experience Contradiction Narrative and Imagination* (pp. 75-95). Adelaide, Australia: Dulwich Centre Publications.

White, M. (1997). *Narratives of Therapists' Lives*. Adelaide, Australia: Dulwich Centre Publications.

Willig, C. (1997). "Making a difference: Can discourse analysis inform psychological interventions?" Paper presented at the Annual Conference of the British Psychological Society, Heriot-Watt University, Edinburgh, April 3-6.

SUGGESTED READINGS

International Journal of Narrative Therapy and Community Work (2002), Number 4. Issue devoted to teaching and supervision.

McKenzie, W. and Monk, G. (1997). Learning and teaching narrative ideas. In G. Monk, J. Winslade, K. Crocket, and D. Epston (Eds.), *Narrative Therapy in Practice: The Archaeology of Hope* (pp. 82-117). San Francisco: Jossey-Bass.

Nightingale, D. and Cromby, J. (1999). *Social Constructionist Psychology: A Critical Analysis of Theory and Practice.* Buckingham, England: Open University Press.

Scaife, J. (1995). *Training to Help: A Survival Guide.* Sheffield, England: Riding Press.

Chapter 13

Storying Counselors: Producing Professional Selves in Supervision

Kathie Crocket

Although a great deal of attention has been paid in recent years to issues of power, knowledge, and relationship in therapy, the literature on these subjects as they pertain to supervision is still remarkably thin. As Kathie Crocket points out in this chapter, much is said about how selves are constituted in conversation, and yet the conversations between "supervisors" and "supervisees" typically construct the former as knowing and seasoned and the latter as unknowing and inexperienced. Crocket suggests that all therapists enter supervision with a good deal of life "expertise," and she is interested in supervision conversations that make room for these knowledges. In effect, supervision becomes a site where therapists may consolidate their professional identities through the expression of their "author-ity."

In this chapter, Crocket takes a critical look at the developmental metaphor that predominates in the counselor supervision literature, arguing that it constructs an unhelpful story of counselors as underdeveloped in their work. She shares a wealth of reflective questions she poses to counselors in training in order to invite them to connect with their own knowledges. The chapter also includes reconstructed conversations that provide a glimpse into her supervision approach.

INTRODUCTION

Counseling supervision is a place for the telling and retelling of stories. Client stories enter the room via video or audio tapes, or they appear in the form of a retelling by counselors. These client stories are told as counselors relate the narrative of their work with clients, and this retelling undergoes a further transformation as supervisors engage with it and coconstruct meaning with counselors through the unfolding supervision conversation. This chapter provides some ideas about how to work with these many stories in a manner that is *productive*. More specifically, it looks at how supervisors and counselors can draw on a multiplicity of rich narratives in supervision to invite forward counselors' professional stories, thus promoting author-ity on the part of counselors through supervision conversations (Crocket, 1999a). Earlier chapters have articulated some practices of respectful therapy, which aims to privilege clients' voices. Taking the position that in many ways supervision and therapy have more in common than much of the current supervision literature allows (compare Carroll, 1996; Gardner, Bobele, and Biever, 1997; Holbway, 1995), I suggest that the ideas and practices of those chapters can also help us think about supervision. If as counselors we commit ourselves to producing respectful relations with our counseling clients and their families, with our agencies and professional associations, why would we stop short of the supervision relationship?

This chapter is based on the constructionist premise that as people story their lives, they also perform and produce their lives. In supervision, then, the stories we tell of our practices and the ethics of those practices do not merely *reflect* our work, they produce us as practitioners and produce our practices. In this chapter, I will render this process visible by referring to supervision as a site of the production of our professional selves. The metaphor of storying, introduced by White and Epston (1989), offers important tools for making sense of supervision in this way. It draws attention to the acts of storying and the persons producing the stories. And it reminds us that we do not tell just any stories: we are dependent upon the cultural stories that are available to us in the production of our personal and professional lives. With that interest, in this chapter I propose enlarging the emphasis, in supervision, on the counselor as an agent producing therapeutic (and supervision) practice, generating possibilities for practice in the dialogue of supervision, and thereby storying his or her professional life.

COUNSELOR AUTHOR-ITY IN SUPERVISION

Although there is a good deal written about the supervision relationship—Holloway (1995), for example, has it at the core of her model—I suggest that counselor author-ity is for the most part neglected in the supervision literature (Crocket, 1999b). The notion of author-ity is derived from the narrative metaphor, which offers up the idea of storying lives. When we story our lives, we take up positions as authors of those stories. In positions of author-ity, we notice the accounts available to us as we story our lives and select those accounts we prefer. This view of counselors as authors of their practice is virtually absent in the literature. Typically, the supervision relationship is depicted in such a way that counselors are produced as people to be acted *upon* in supervision: to be developed, to be subject to assessment and appropriate intervention, to have their practice monitored and evaluated. Counselors are thus found in subjected positions in most accounts of supervision (Crocket, 1999b). In contrast, I am interested in counselors as *actors* in supervision, as agents producing therapeutic practice as they engage in the to and fro of supervision conversations. Although some attention has been paid to advising supervisors about collaborative supervision relationships (for example, Anderson and Swim, 1995), I think that we need to go further than this and to prepare counselors to be collaborative partners in supervision. Put differently, I am interested in counselors as story*ing,* rather than stor*ied,* in supervision.

In my work as a counselor educator, I attend to this storying aspect of supervision at the beginning of our counselor education program. In inviting counseling students to think about the positions-in-relation that may be offered them in supervision, distinguishing between subjected positions that do not privilege their own voices and subjective ones that do. I am interested in helping them identify positions that will be most productive of their agency as counselors—that will promote their professional author-ity. In one of the teaching sessions as part of this work of orientation to supervision, I invite counseling students into an imaginary storying experience. As we begin, I ask them to think of someone, from another setting, who knows them and their work or their qualities well. They might think of one of the people who supported their application to our program, a professional colleague in a previous setting, someone with whom they work on a committee, or a friend who supports their current study. I then ask them to imagine that individual having a conversation with the person who is to be their supervisor. As they imagine this conversation, I ask a range of reflexive questions that invite them to inhabit the scenarios being asked about. (As readers, you might like to read these questions aloud: they may be easier to engage with that way.)

- What might this former colleague tell your supervisor about the qualities he or she most appreciates in you and your work?
- What ways of being do you think this person might want to speak of appreciating as he or she speaks of his or her experiences of you? What experiences of you will he or she be drawing on in this telling?
- As you imagine this conversation, what might your former colleague tell your supervisor about what he or she thinks your supervisor might come to appreciate about working with you, in supervision?
- As you imagine yourself entering the supervision relationship with your supervisor, what will it be like for you entering that supervision relationship, carrying with you these accounts of yourself that you have just overheard in this imagined conversation?
- How do you see yourself as you engage in the work of supervision alongside your supervisor? What does it mean for you to see yourself in these ways? What does it mean for the supervision relationship that you see yourself in these ways?
- How do you see your supervisor seeing you? What does it mean for you and for the supervisor that you see your supervisor seeing you in these ways? What does it mean for the work of supervision?

Questions such as these open the supervision space to be something other than an assumed hierarchy of expert and beginner. The questions offer counselors positions where they, too, are seen to bring experiences, wisdom, and valued personal and professional qualities and experiences to supervision. In this way they are positioned to engage in robust reflection on their counseling work in supervision. My experience has been that these acts of imagination work to position counselors well, too, to engage in building a working supervision relationship in collaboration with their supervisors. They are less likely to find themselves in the position of having supervision *done to* them.

Students have spoken of the value of making more visible to themselves the many stories that make up their lives at a time when a story of themselves as a beginning counselor might obscure the richness of what they already bring for the work of supervision. These questions are not just for beginners, however. More experienced colleagues have also found it useful at the time of beginning a new supervision relationship to think about how they want to introduce themselves to their new supervisor, and what accounts of themselves they wish to be productive of their professional selves as they enter that working relationship. Who are we, as we sit down together, you and I, in supervision? What stories of our personal and professional lives do we both bring to this work? The pause in which we ask these questions offers us space to think about respectful relationship in supervision, relationship that recognizes that we are multiply storied. This emphasis on multivocality—many stories, many voices—contrasts with a well-entrenched narrative of counselors as "developing"—an account that presumes a progressive unfolding according to arbitrarily specified norms for counselor competence.

SOME PROBLEMS
WITH DEVELOPMENTAL ASSUMPTIONS

As I pay attention to an account of supervision that makes room for a story of the resourcefulness that counselors bring to supervision, I note that those accounts of supervision which obscure such resourcefulness are so familiar that they are often taken for granted and their strategies not noticed. In my experience, those accounts depend upon the developmental metaphor and they persist sometimes even in places where their presence might be less taken for granted. Writing in the context of developmental psychology, Burman (1994) noted that developmental accounts become "naturalized": their constructs are taken to represent reality. Despite warnings such as Holloway's (1987) that the attractiveness of developmental supervision models might obscure the need for rigorous investigation of these models, developmental constructions have been naturalized in many accounts of and in everyday understandings of supervision. Naturalized, developmental constructions contribute to an idea that has persisted even in some accounts of a postmodern practice of supervision. This idea suggests that the storying of professional identity is somewhat problematic in supervision because counselors early in their careers do not have enough knowledge or experience to draw on in that storying. The idea was expressed in two important supervision texts. Gardner, Bobele, and Biever (1997) suggested that while in postmodern therapy there is an assumption of clients being experts on their own lives, there is not the assumption in supervision that counselors are "experts on therapy" (p. 224). Their point was echoed by Bernard and Goodyear (1998) who, writing about narrative approaches in supervision, suggested that trainees are "just beginning" to develop stories of "self-as-professional" while clients have "well developed" stories (p. 22). Both author teams thus draw a distinction between therapy clients, whose knowing and expertise about their lives is to be valued, and counselors in supervision who, they propose, come without material to be storied because of a thinness of *professional* experience. I believe that to suggest there is little material to draw on in storying the professional identity of a counselor new to the field is to edit out the possibility that the counselor brings a richness of *lived* experience upon which they draw as they story their professional identity. I believe that the storying of professional identity that we do in the supervision room depends upon very much more than just stories about therapy that come from the profession's knowledge stores. Rather, supervision might be practiced as a site for bringing forth the values, ideas, and histories that all counselors bring to their work (see White, 1997), and thus for producing new possibilities for effective and ethical practice. Of course professional knowledge and wisdom and practice experience is to be valued. However, it is not all that there is, and the field is impoverished if we behave in supervision as if it is.

MULTIPLE VOICES: PRODUCING POSSIBILITIES FOR PRACTICE

The storying of our professional lives is an active and ongoing process that unfolds through talk: the talk of therapeutic conversations and the talk *about* that talk, which occurs in counseling supervision. The following conversation is a reconstruction of the many reflective exchanges I am involved in through the practice of supervision. It illustrates the ways in which counselor author-ity is produced by inviting multiple voices into the conversation—including not only the voice of the counselor but also the voice of the client. Ultimately our work should be accountable to the persons with whom we work; by inviting their voices into supervision conversations, we assist counselors in producing their work in accordance with their ethical commitment to clients.

COUNSELOR: Do you remember the time you interviewed me on tape about my work with Maureen? I'd been so determined to support her in the struggle against agoraphobia but it seemed that we were no longer making any headway. Sure, there'd been change, but she was still caught in an oppressive marriage relationship that seemed to be restraining further change, and it seemed that there was nowhere else for the counseling to go. Perhaps this was going to be as good as it was going to get for Maureen. I was losing hope. Your idea of bringing forth values made a difference to me then. You suggested we videotape a record of my work with Maureen as seen through my eyes. You interviewed me about the work so that I could kind of take stock. Making a taped record of this made a sense to me: I wanted Maureen to hear what I'd say. Our supervision wasn't just about you and me. More than merely taking stock with you of this work, I wanted to keep Maureen in authority over the value of the work we were doing. What would she say about these hard-won gains that I'd been thinking were not enough?

SUPERVISOR: Once you invited Maureen into the conversation, as it were, you began to see things differently. We began the interview having agreed that we'd review your understanding of what Maureen had sought consultation with you about, and the ground she had gained so far, so that you could take the tape back to Maureen and consult her about your understandings.

COUNSELOR: As I told the story of our counseling work together, my respect for Maureen, both in her resilience in the struggle and for the steps she had taken to make things different for herself, became more visible to me. The telling brought forth the regard I had for her. The sense of Maureen being with us in the supervision room as I told our story was productive of that respect. I became more and more interested to know what Maureen might have wanted to say had she been there. In the care of telling the story, I came to appreciate more deeply the significance of the work we'd done together and of the steps Maureen had taken to win some difference in her life.

SUPERVISOR: You took the tape to your next counseling session with Maureen and played the conversation we'd had.

COUNSELOR: Yes, and one of the most important things I learned from that was how easily we can take for granted what our respect offers our clients. As Maureen listened to the tape of me telling you her story, she heard a story of her life from a new position. The grip of isolation was further broken as we listened together.

Joining with counselors in the production of their author-ity includes facilitating conversations that enable them to "hear" the voices of the persons with whom they are working. At times, it may also mean bringing to the surface of the supervision conversation voices in the background of that conversation: the cultural discourses that provide the life support for the problems clients encounter.

COUNSELOR: I remember wondering if the changes Sally had been making would endure. She'd been doing so well. Was it possible that she'd won that much ground back from bulimia when it had had such a hold? What would we do next in the therapy to make the most of these changes? Could I trust that we really had gained ground, and in what ways might I be blind to bulimia's sneaky tricks? What come-back tactics might bulimia have up its sleeve? That was what I was asking in supervision.

SUPERVISOR: I remember your delight in the ground Sally had won and your desire to shore those gains up. I asked you then if I might interview you as bulimia: given the uncertainty you were expressing, I asked you if you were interested to get bulimia's view on things.

COUNSELOR: Your first question opened the flood gates. You said, "Bulimia, has the therapy in any way taken you by surprise?" It turned out I had plenty to say about that. I really did think bulimia had been taken by surprise, because Sally and I had made such a thorough investigation of its tactics. I could see more clearly how the ground Sally had won wasn't due to chance, and wasn't too much at risk, as we'd been so thorough in unpacking the problem and Sally was so clear about what she now wanted. bulimia didn't have too many places left to hide. I saw we'd identified bulimia's blind spots and Sally was indeed gaining the upper hand. Then you asked me what might happen next in the therapy that would give me, as bulimia, cause for concern.

SUPERVISOR: You took on the voice of bulimia, in that interview. How that was helpful?

COUNSELOR: Well, there's always more than one story, and more than one position from which a story can be told. As a counselor, I'd been so delighted to share with Sally as she reclaimed her life. I knew she was feeling pleased, but I was still worried. When I spoke as bulimia, it gave me another vantage point from which to look at the scene. Speaking with the voice of bulimia didn't resolve the problems it invited, but it offered me a richer understanding of bulimia's workings and of the dimensions of the work Sally and I were doing together. And I went back to the next meeting with Sally and asked her what she thought about her and I inviting bulimia into the counseling room for an interview. Different voices make different conversations possible.

SHARING THE CLOAK: RELATIONAL RESPONSIBILITY IN SUPERVISION

A noteworthy feature of the preceding conversations is that they are not oriented toward monitoring clinical performance. Instead, they are generative conversations that invite the many voices of both counselors and their clients into the supervision session. In so doing, these conversations create space for counselors to produce responsible professional practice, rather than establishing a context for the supervisor to take responsibility for the "junior" counselor. And so these conversations are not principally oriented toward checking on the "assessment" the counselors had done at the outset of their work, or gathering details of their "treatment plan." This is not to suggest that eating disorders are not complex and challenging problems; however, I prefer to make at least as much space for the voices of clients as for the regulatory bodies that prescribe narrow modes of practice. Supervision is about producing quality assurance of effective and ethical therapeutic practice. Supervision ultimately is for the client. I do not believe Sally or Maureen would opt for an interrogation of her counselor's assessment and treatment plans at the expense of the preceding conversations.

This is not to say that there is no place for a "quality assurance" role in supervision. However, I believe we may actually sacrifice that quality if the profession diminishes counselors' responsibility—their agency, their author-ity—by having supervisors assume full responsibility on their behalf. I have often heard counselors reflect on their early experiences as counselors in supervision, when it seemed that there was little space left for them to be responsible for their own practice because so much responsibility was taken up by the supervisor. There was little room for them to grapple with ethical questions, for example, when the answers were already being presented, almost before counselors could ask themselves the questions.

As a supervisor, I do not wish to abdicate responsibility, but I look to *share* it with counselors. After all, if they are to be in a position to share responsibility with clients in the therapy room, I need to share it with them in the supervision room. I think that when I make space in the supervision room for a counselor's capacities to be seen by us both, I can have more assurance that they are producing themselves in ethical ways. When a supervisor wears a cloak of responsibility that covers the work of counselors, too, it can obscure their capacities, and the voice of their knowledges. That cloak can act as a burden that renders supervisors unavailable to an understanding of what counselor and supervisor might produce together, squandering the generative potential of supervision conversations.

I am interested in using supervision as a forum for enlarging the capacities of counselors for knowing and acting, working with counselors to produce them as agents in their work. This way of working produces a different power relation, one that is productive of relational responsibility, and that includes responsibility to (rather than for) clients.

STORIES FOR ACTION: THE WORK OF SUPERVISION

There are many stories that produce the work of supervision. As supervisors, we are in a privileged position to determine which stories will be heard and which obscured. Too often a professional or regulatory story obscures many other potentially generative narratives in supervision. This chapter has offered some ideas and examples of supervision conversations that make room for the voices of counselors, clients, and even problems, to create a space for counselors to produce responsible and ethical practice in accordance with their own situated author-ity. That author-ity is situated in work with clients, in the values and histories that have produced counselors' lives, as well as in professional knowledges. In many respects, these ideas are about applying to supervision the possibility-generating, competence-oriented practices which are hallmarks of respectful postmodern therapeutic practice.

REFERENCES

Anderson, H. and Swim, S. (1995). Supervision as collaborative conversation: Connecting the voices of supervisor and supervisee. *Journal of Systemic Therapies* *14*(2): 1-13.

Bernard, J. M. and Goodyear, R. K. (1998). *Fundamentals of clinical supervision.* Needham Heights, MA: Allyn and Bacon.

Burman, E. (1994). *Deconstructing developmental psychology.* London: Routledge.

Carroll, M. (1996). *Counseling supervision: Theory, skills and practice.* London: Cassell.

Crocket, K. (1999a). Supervision: A site of authority production. *New Zealand Journal of Counseling* 20: 75-83; Errata (2000), *New Zealand Journal of Counseling* 21: 85-87.

Crocket, K. (1999b). Supervision: What kind of working alliance is it? In *Proceedings of New Zealand Association of Counselors 25th Conference: A place to stand* (pp. 181-187). Hamilton, New Zealand: Waikato Branch, New Zealand Association of Counsellors.

Gardner, G. L, Bobele, M., and Biever, J. L. (1997). Postmodern models of family therapy supervision. In T. C. Todd and C. L. Storm (Eds.), *The complete systemic supervisor: Context, philosophy, and pragmatics* (pp. 217-228). Boston: Allyn & Bacon.

Holloway, E. L. (1987). Developmental models of supervision: Is it development? *Professional Psychology Research and Practice* 18: 203-216.

Holloway, E. L. (1995). *Clinical supervision: A systems approach.* Thousand Oaks, CA: Sage.

White, M. (1997). *Narratives of therapists' lives.* Adelaide, Australia: Dulwich Centre.

White, M. and Epston, D. (1989). *Literate means to therapeutic ends.* Adelaide, Australia: Dulwich Centre.

SUGGESTED READINGS

Fine, M. and Turner, J. (1997). Collaborative supervision: Minding the power. In T. C. Todd and C. L. Storm (Eds.), *The complete systemic supervisor: Context, philosophy, and pragmatics* (pp. 229-240). Boston: Allyn & Bacon.

White, M. (1997). *Narratives of therapists' lives.* Adelaide, Australia: Dulwich Centre.

Chapter 14

Power, Gender, and Accountability in Supervision

Heather Gridley

Heather Gridley's chapter offers a unique and close examination of power issues in supervision from the perspective of gender. It draws on the author's research into a feminist model of supervision for women psychologists, asking how it is possible to minimize relational violence in the supervision relationship while guaranteeing accountability and empowerment. As the author states, supervision provides a gatekeeping role and entry point to the profession of psychology and therapy, yet in terms of gender power relationships it tends to be a situation "where women get monitored, men get mentored."

After a review of the literature on power differentials in supervision, Gridley presents a qualitative research project involving four feminist supervisors and their female supervisees. This provides the basis for a feminist re-vision of supervision around themes of nurturance and safety, power, mentoring, accountable practice, and consciousness-raising. The chapter concludes with a challenge to male and female supervisors and supervisees to critically reflect on and make transparent issues of power and gender politics in their practices.

Supervision is an odd term. To the beginning counselor,* the prospect conjures up images of someone looking over your shoulder—indeed, my initial literature search linking gender with supervision unearthed references to prison guards! Michael White prefers the term *covision,* while in the Netherlands the process is described as *intervision.* These alternative terms represent attempts to equalize re-

---

*I have followed the lead of Jeanette Shopland (2000) in using the terms *counselor, therapist,* and *psychotherapist* interchangeably "in a deliberate attempt to subvert the claims to status or relative effectiveness that may accompany these labels" (p. 7).

lationships and minimize power differentials—which is also the focus of this chapter.

Supervision is a process common to most human service professions. The literature suggests that supervision has two basic functions: professional socialization and consumer protection. Professional socialization encompasses development of supervisees via maintenance of their knowledge base, skills enhancement, inculcation of values and attitudes, evaluation of worthiness/readiness for admission to the profession, and support of career prospects—akin to mentoring. Consumer protection involves recognition of new practitioners' limitations, by providing the "safety net" of an experienced practitioner, legally accountable for the supervisee's actions.

This chapter draws on a study examining supervision in the professional training of psychologists, with particular reference to women's location in the discourse and practice of psychology in Australia. Examinations of gender trends in psychology in Australia (Cumming and Hyslop, 1998), the United States and internationally (Denmark, 1998), New Zealand (Lapsley and Wilkinson, 2001), and Britain (Kagan and Lewis, 1990) revealed men's predominance and greater visibility in research, publishing, training, and leadership positions, while practitioners, students, and clients were predominantly female. These trends persist into the twenty-first century, with Australian Psychological Society (APS) membership statistics showing that 31 percent of fellows are women compared with 68 percent of members and 83 percent of student and associate members; moreover, 61 percent of those employed in universities are women compared with 71 percent as practitioners, and even more in the public sector (APS, 2001). However these figures are interpreted, supervisees are increasingly likely to be women.

Feminist analysis offers much to discussions of power and accountability because feminism has always highlighted the operation of power at societal and interpersonal levels, while psychology's reductionist approach has been accused of underestimating or individualizing issues of power (Kitzinger, 1991). This chapter considers supervision in terms of power dynamics and their implications for beginning practitioners and, indirectly, for psychotherapy practice.

HISTORICAL CONTEXT

The history of supervision raises alarm bells in terms of gender and power. Supervision theory dates from the late nineteenth century, when women began being widely recruited as teachers. Slack (1990) cites Payne's (1873) major work on supervision, regarding the relative fitness of men and women to manage schools:

> Reasoning from fact, we may learn from the many families left in charge by women . . . that woman unaided, is not equal to the task . . . while the known instincts of woman which prompt her to act from feeling, rather than from deliberate purpose, will lead us to expect a weakness, requiring the supervision of a man. (Slack, 1990, p. 3)

This resonates with Chernesky's (1986) observation a century later regarding the patriarchal nature of social work supervision that "when the predominant gender of the workforce is female, the use of supervision to keep workers dependent and submissive is more likely" (p. 136).

Slack (1990) observed how the languages of religion and science together invested supervision with overtones of divine, patriarchal power, evident in its root meaning, "seeing over," and its common explication as "supervision." Slack warned that "one needs to go beyond defining supervision as a truth or technique to supervision as a relational process involving historical metaphors of power" (p. 8). There has been little comparable deconstruction of counseling supervision, a notable exception being Hawkins and Shohet's (2000) textbook, which introduces a triangular representation of power dynamics in transcultural supervision.

A second power-related concern emerges from the fact that supervision was originally appropriated by the new social-science-based human service professions in their quest for acceptance alongside established disciplines such as science and professions such as law and medicine. Since "expert" professions and their scientific knowledge claims have been heavily critiqued (e.g., Illich et al., 1977; Brown, 1997; John, 1998), the question remains: how empowering to clients is an activity in which a counselor and supervisor discuss their problems in the clients' absence?

These two cautionary notes embedded in the history of supervision mirror two present-day sources of contention concerning power. One relates to implications for supervisees, and the other to accountability to clients. Because the study under discussion here focused on the supervision relationship, I am mainly concerned with the first issue, but it is essential to keep coming back to clients as the intended primary beneficiaries of supervision, whether or not they participate in or even know about the process.

MENTORING OR MONITORING?

It might be said that where women get monitored, men get mentored. Whereas supervision began as a means of monitoring and controlling women's entry to a profession, mentoring was almost entirely associated with men's career development (e.g., Levinson et al., 1978). Since most definitions of mentoring specify one-to-one relationships between more experienced and less experienced persons, the overlap with supervision is clear. But what is absent from discussions of mentoring is the emphasis on quality control and evaluation central to supervision. Thus the flavor of mentoring discourses is of initiation of the select few into an elite and relatively fixed hierarchy, with scant attention to mentees' responsibilities, for example, to behave ethically or be accountable to clients and the wider community.

The benefits of mentorship as applied to supervision are confirmed in career development studies urging early establishment of mentor-protégé relationships, since supervisors discussing their own mentors ascribed greatest importance to the first (Burke and McKeen, 1990). These stuides recommend specific mentoring behaviors, such as maintaining an open-door policy, inclusion in informal networks, verbal support and encouragement, and one-to-one counseling and discussion.

When mentoring is promoted as an equal employment opportunity tool, the emphasis usually is on ensuring a critical mass of appropriately mentored women or minority group members, rather than on structural change to organizations or institutions perpetuating inequality. If professional traditions and world views to be passed on are presented as indisputable truths, the very nature of supervision lessens the likelihood that recipients of such "truths" will question their validity.

Historically, mentoring has served to protect privilege. Supervision monitors the performance of aspirants at a profession's entrance gates. The fact that mentoring has mostly been accessed by men in male-dominated organizations and activities (McCormick, 1991), while supervision is more commonly associated with stereotypically female professions, represents a challenge for counseling professions, whose ethos has been predominantly male driven, yet whose clients have largely been and whose composition increasingly is female. Can women access the individual and collective benefits of mentoring without succumbing to its individualistic, patriarchal overtones? Can the monitoring function traditionally implied in the supervision of subordinates be transformed into an accountability clause in the predominantly self-serving nature of mentoring? Does a supportive induction of women into counseling professions necessarily render practice more accountable to (women) clients in general?

CONSTRUCTIONS OF POWER IN SUPERVISION

When practitioners speak of "getting myself some supervision" as a buffer to the demands of frontline work, they anticipate a freely contracted, benevolent arrangement of demonstrable benefit to the practitioner, the agency, and ultimately the client. The salience of power differentials may not immediately be apparent.

Several studies have illustrated the operation of power differentials in supervision. Huber (1991) compared job evaluations completed by incumbents with those completed by their workplace supervisors. Incumbents rated their own performance higher than did supervisors, yet lowered their ratings more to reach consensus than supervisors raised theirs. Dixon and Claiborn (1987) proposed a social influence model as an alternative to traditional developmental and learning models of counselor supervision, but overlooked the ethical uses or potential abuses of the supervisor's ascribed social power.

Nelson and Holloway (1990) undertook a microanalysis of supervision and found macrolevel implications. They found that both male and female supervisors (and their female supervisees) were subject to socially constructed, gendered expectations of expertise and power operating, largely unconsciously, to obstruct the assumption of power by females. The cumulative impact of such disparities is a likely factor in the relative absence, documented earlier, of women in the upper echelons of the profession.

Power differentials affect both parties' decisions regarding their degree of self-disclosure and the blurring or maintaining of boundaries between supervision, therapy, and friendship. Such decisions remain largely the prerogative of the supervisor, underlining the imbalance of power even in apparently egalitarian supervision arrangements.

Feminist social work training and supervision literature emerged in the mid-1980s, promoting egalitarian alternatives to traditional hierarchical models (Crossan, 1986; Travers, 1986). They emphasized power sharing, reciprocity, shared learning, and an action orientation as characteristic of supervision provided by feminists. Their suggestions included contracting out evaluation components of supervision, and introducing consciousness-raising groups: "Learning should be a joint venture between teacher and taught, providing space for women together to develop their sense of personal and political power" (Marchant and Wearing, 1986, p. 205). This resonates with McWhirter's (1998) notion of empowerment in counselor education as maintaining responsive systems for integrating student input and attending to student concerns while incorporating wider support for the empowerment of others.

Some theorists question attempts to equalize hierarchical relationships such as supervision. Avoiding the realities of power dynamics, whether structurally or individually located, is considered naïve (Squire, 1990; Perkins, 1991). McWhirter (1998) supports collaborative approaches aimed at reducing the hierarchical nature of teaching and supervisory relationships, but cautions against obfuscating "the very real power differences that exist between counselor and client, faculty member and student" (p. 15). Supervisors in education, licensing, or professional registration contexts retain an evaluative, gatekeeping function that is at odds with any supportive, developmental, or collegiate roles they might prefer to establish. The assumption that power differentials always need to be minimized (and disappear altogether in same-sex relationships) is questionable in the context of supervision.

THE PROJECT

Two functions are typically ascribed to supervision: professional socialization or gatekeeping and consumer protection. Both are problematic: the former for its elitist, conservative implications and the latter for its paternalistic and paradoxical assumptions that consumers require protection via processes that remain beyond their awareness, consent, or control. Yet these constitute the two aspects of supervision most open to reconstruction from a feminist perspective. Thus professional socialization might become mentoring and consciousness raising while consumer protection might be reframed as accountability.

Consideration of gender and power relationships in supervision led me to ask: how might a feminist model of supervision look, and what happens to the supervisory relationship and process when the supervisor (and perhaps the supervisee) identifies herself as a feminist?

Four supervisors identified as feminist psychologists were recruited via the APS Women and Psychology Interest Group, along with their supervisees. All were women. Given the exploratory nature of the research, to investigate feminist supervision in practice and uncover the theory implicit in it, a qualitative approach was chosen. Supervisors' and supervisees' focus groups were videotaped, as were supervision sessions with each pair. At a final review session, edited segments of videotape selected by the pairs were presented for discussion. Tapes were transcribed and data was analyzed thematically. The research process itself was designed to meet feminist goals such as articulating values, consciousness raising, empowering participants, and promoting change.

The individuals in the supervision relationship discussed below are a composite of the pairs in the project—quotes are drawn, with permission, from participants' comments, but altered sufficiently to preserve anonymity. The names are pseudonyms.

Kim is a forty-two-year-old former teacher who completed her psychology training after raising two children. She is accumulating her mandatory two years of supervised experience by working part-time in a student counseling service, and also as a volunteer with a telephone crisis line. Maria is an experienced counseling psychologist active in women's groups within and outside the profession.

FINDINGS AND DISCUSSION

The experiences reported by all participants confirmed that supervision has significant implications for those entering counseling professions. Predominant themes emerging from the data analysis were:

1. the centrality of the supervision relationship in terms of nurturance and safety for women supervisees;
2. the importance of addressing, rather than denying or attempting to neutralize, power and gender issues within the supervision process;
3. the role of the supervisor as mentor in the professional development of the supervisee;
4. the potential within supervision for consciousness raising and an action orientation.

What follows are some practice examples of each of these themes, drawing on the composite supervisory experiences of Kim and Maria.

Nurturance and Safety in the Supervision Relationship

KIM: You don't have to play a role—here I am as me—I've never had that experience before, even from females . . . I want to go on, and I've got to go with who I am.

MARIA: You go through a period of learning where the beginning is involved with doubts . . . I guess I'm making an argument for a road where you don't lose yourself.

Here the focus was on Kim's own career development and her experience of supervision as nurturing her aspirations. Kim's reflection that her current supervision experience was atypical highlights the limited capacity of "good ordinary" supervision to attend to women supervisees. All participants made some reference to nurturance and "a safe environment" as primary needs of women in supervision. "I feel comfortable to acknowledge that I'm trying to cope with two kids and a career as well—others might say, if you can't cope, get out." In contrast, Kim's academic supervisor had seen her as a dilettante, studying psychology as a hobby: "I felt apologetic for taking up a place at my age."

Referring to a training exercise in her workplace, Kim describes supervision as "creating a safe space, an equal relationship—in the space they created between them, things happen."

Power—The Supervisor As Gatekeeper/Monitor

KIM: I sit in a different chair for supervision! You give up your power—and that's compounded if the supervisor doesn't respond.

MARIA: I'm never late for my supervisor, but I'm often late for my supervisee—that's a power issue.

Mainstream models of supervision make minimal reference to power differentials between supervisor and supervisee or to the wider structural differentials between men and women in patriarchal societies. In contrast, feminist approaches often emphasize power as something to be neutralized via egalitarian forms of supervision (and therapy). Participants in this project appeared to go further, and were actively engaged in attempts to make overt and to understand the nature of power as integral to supervision.

As Kim and Maria discuss the limits to equality in therapy, there are parallels with similar issues in their own relationship. In supervision, Kim gives the example of a client having almost called her one weekend to invite her to a film: "We need to keep in mind the power balance—I'm responsible for watching that, I'm the one trained to be aware of it—then I wonder if I've been overdoing the boundary setting on something as simple as friendship between women?" Maria's response invites Kim to consider in which role she is more useful to her client at present: "Oh, as a therapist, definitely," replies Kim. The example has parallels within their own relationship. As Kim's supervision contract nears its end, she considers extending it beyond the mandatory two years. Maria, not wishing to lock Kim into a permanently needful position, suggests that supervision be formally terminated, and that they arrange to meet henceforth as colleagues. Kim reflects in retrospect: "Maria started quite methodically from being more in control to more equalizing during supervision—now we're friends." Although not everyone would consider friendship a desirable outcome of supervision, the interactions between Kim and Maria ensure that power issues are not overlooked.

Even within the apparently affirming supervision relationships displayed in this project, some self-deprecation is implied by participants' references to supervisors as "fairy godmothers" who give "permission to be what I thought was impossible," "control the process," and have "more skills than me." Of course, what some might conceptualize negatively as dependency, others might consider a vital and nurturing supportive relationship, questioning whether the "masculine" ideal of rugged independence is always a healthy goal.

"A lot of what we do works to level what we do—but the supervisor has the ultimate power to decide the level of equality" (Maria). Rather than ignoring the power differentials inherent in supervision, participants acknowledged their operation. One supervisee welcomed the supervisor's power to control the process during her probationary period, while a supervisor emphasized "the way you use the power you have," and another acknowledged that power also involves responsibility.

"I think it was a power issue he has with women . . . I was treated like a nincompoop and so I behaved like one . . . he wasn't allowing this uppity woman any leeway at all" (Kim, in reference to her academic supervisor). It was the supervisees who were most conscious of power dynamics and who spent more time on this issue in their focus group than the supervisors, confirming the tendency of the more powerful to minimize their power and deny the nature of their privilege. The supervisees' greater awareness of power differentials within supervision, and the hints of dependency implied in some of their comments, underscore a need for ongoing vigilance to offset the profession's traditional understating of such issues while continuing to operate within a discourse and set of structures steeped in power and control.

The bottom line is that current professional certification requirements place supervisors firmly, if sometimes reluctantly, in the role of monitoring supervisees' performance and gatekeeping their entry to the profession. It seems unrealistic and unhelpful to pretend that supervision involves a cozy, equal, dyadic relationship with no reference to the wider structures that determine its limits. McWhirter (1998) concurs, cautioning against any pretense of equality "as if all involved are equally free to present their viewpoints and to initiate change" (p. 15).

The Supervisor As Mentor

MARIA: My agenda is to support other women in the profession.

KIM: I have a collection of mentors, four really strong women—I call them my four fairy godmothers! I ask myself, how would this or that one approach a particular problem I have.

All participants referred in some way to the contribution of supervision in their early career survival, and to having observed the behavior of their supervisor(s) and used it as a model. "The people ahead of you have a big influence—we are setting up role models for ourselves all the time."

In their focus group, supervisees referred to "things we like and love about our supervisors," as well as to valuable information, support, and resources provided by them. The practical consequences of Maria's stated agenda are noted by Kim, who valued her women supervisors as strong, confident women with a sense of humor, whose example "gave me permission to be what I thought was impossible; what *could be* then came to pass—they were a mirror for me to model myself on."

As noted earlier, there is some danger in an uncritical acceptance of mentoring as a weapon in women counselors' onslaught on the profession's "glass ceiling." But despite fears that it merely socializes a select few into the professional status quo, critics such as McCormick (1991) argue for the transformation rather than eradication of mentoring, "since the evidence so clearly indicates the necessity of having a mentor" (p. 5). Within the helping professions, mentoring may be useful, but supervision is usually mandatory at some stage, strengthening the argument for transformatory mentorship functions.

"I've had wonderful peer supervision—that's my real supervision experience . . . sought out for specific purposes: mutual trust, egalitarian, safety—I assume that's what I'd be providing—a safe environment—is that feminist?" (Maria). Maria's reflection highlights one way in which concerns about one-to-one supervision fostering dependency in supervisees can be offset—by spreading supervisory functions and promoting peer group consultation (Chernesky, 1986). Each year the APS Women and Psychology Interest Groups in Melbourne and Sydney conduct sessions on "Getting started as women in psychology" as a means of collective mentoring for beginning practitioners.

Accountability and Consciousness Raising

MARIA: I'm not into overservicing [of clients]—it's a matter of being open to further contact without giving the message that once you're here, you come forever.

KIM: She kept bringing in the bigger picture, the community context.

Here the focus was on the content of supervision—how Maria and Kim used supervision to promote emancipatory counseling practices—the litmus test of feminist supervision as distinct from mainstream supervision. Reworking accountability to incorporate sociopolitical context impacts directly on the supervision process and indirectly on the supervisee's developing praxis. Although mainstream models emphasize consumer protection as a reason for controlling entry to the profession, such controls are often designed more to protect the interests of the profession itself by restricting competition and enhancing the mystique of expert power.

Reworking consumer protection's paternalistic "on behalf of" overtones demands an accountability where the consumer is judge of whose interests are being met and a recognition of the limits to therapy as "the answer." Sherman (1984) questions the likelihood of counselors acting as social change agents, and suggests that any initiatives must begin with a recognition of the ways in which the role, training, and values of the counselor "limit possibilities for fundamental change" (p. 112). McWhirter (1998) advocates the development of contextual awareness, critical consciousness, and community activism within her model of counselor education, "embracing the notion that counseling can be, and often is, a vehicle of oppression" (p. 24).

In this project, the contents of all taped sessions reveal an awareness of "the way culture and patriarchy affect what's happened" (Maria). One supervisor compares the "reductionist viewpoint" with a need for "opening out," while another's approach to counseling is framed in terms of balancing support with choice in offering services. Maria and Kim's taped session is devoted to a woman-sensitive review of Kim's counseling practice, simultaneously affirming her initiatives and those of her clients. Within the demanding field of sexual-assault counseling, an action orientation offers one antidote to the burnout experienced by workers constantly confronted with evidence of traumatic oppression. Supervision that encompasses such "big picture" involvement as Reclaim the Night marches and rape-law reform can be affirming for the practitioner seeking channels for her accumulating rage. "It's not just sympathy for women's issues, it's understanding that they're political, structural."

CONCLUSION

A re-visioning of supervision must recognize that choices are constructed within and constrained by structures and discourses surrounding individual participants, and that the necessarily unequal position of any supervisee is compounded if she is a woman. The possibilities raised here—group supervision, an action orientation, and a notion of empowerment as a collective, outward-looking process rather than a singular, active verb—underscore the transformatory potential of supervision for the profession.

The study discussed here introduced a feminist perspective to supervision as a means of addressing inequities within psychology and inadequacies in its practice. Having a feminist supervisor appeared to benefit supervisees. Whether such benefits rendered their practice more accountable is not so clear. Implications for both women and men in psychotherapeutic practice include the potential of mentoring as a tool for changing professional cultures as well as promoting the development of individual therapists and the importance of overting and understanding power in the supervision agenda. Supervision can provide a positive springboard for change directed backward into preservice training, upward into the infrastructures of professional self-interest, and outward to clients and communities. In the spirit of critical self-reflection, I invite supervisors and supervisees to consider the following questions:

For Supervisors

- Where do your politics sit within your approach to supervision?
- How would you explain your style to potential supervisees?
- What would you ask them?

For Supervisees

- How would you go about interviewing prospective supervisors?
- What would you (not) want them to know about you?

For Both

- How do you see gender, culture, or politics impacting on your choice of supervisor/supervisee, and on the supervision process? What might a feminist-informed supervision contract entail?
- How would you describe your relationship with your supervisor/supervisee—strictly professional? equal? friendly? What would be more comfortable (and/or challenging!) for you?
- In what ways does power operate in your supervisory relationship(s)?
- In what ways might a supervisor act as mentor or role model in the career development of a supervisee? Are there "downsides" to such terms?
- How do you negotiate the limits to your relationship?
- What issues have arisen in supervision that might benefit from a critical or sociopolitical analysis?
- Have you dealt with anything in supervision that was not or could not be addressed in preservice training?
- Is there any difference between (a) a feminist supervisor, (b) a woman supervisor, and (c) any good supervisor? In other words, would you attribute your approach to experience of supervision to gender, politics, personality, or training? Do they ever conflict?
- How does your supervision address the question of accountability to clients?

REFERENCES

Australian Psychological Society (2001). *Annual Report.* Melbourne Australian Psychological Society Publications.

Brown, L. (1997). Ethics in Psychology: *Cui bono?* In D. Fox and I. Prilleltensky (Eds.), *Critical Psychology: An Introduction* (pp. 51-67). London: Sage.

Burke, R.J. and McKeen, C.A. (1990). Mentoring in organizations: Implications for women. *Journal of Business Ethics 9:* 317-332.

Chernesky, R.H. (1986). A new model of supervision. In N. Van den Bergh and L.B. Cooper (Eds.), *Feminist Visions for Social Work* (pp. 128-148). Silver Spring, MA: National Association of Social Workers.

Crossan, D. (1986). "Feminism and social work supervision." Unpublished paper, Wellington, NZ.

Cumming, G. and Hyslop, W. (1998). Professional training in psychology and academic staff profiles in Australian universities. *Australian Psychologist 33:* 62-67.

Denmark, F.L. (1998). Women and psychology: An international perspective. *American Psychologist 53:* 465-473

Dixon, D.N. and Claiborn, C.D. (1987). A social influence approach to counselor supervision. In J. Maddux, C. Stoltenberg, and R. Rosenwein (Eds.), *Social Processes in Clinical and Counseling Psychology* (pp. 83-93). New York: Springer-Verlag.

Hawkins, P. and Shohet, R. (2000). *Supervision in the Helping Professions* (Second Edition). Buckingham, UK: Open University Press.

Huber, V. (1991). Comparison of supervisor-incumbent and male-female multidimensional job evaluation ratings. *Journal of Applied Psychology 76:* 115-121.

Illich, I., Zola, I., McKnight, J., Caplan, J., and Shaiken, H. (1977). *Disabling Professions: Ideas in Progress Open Forum.* London: Marion Rogers.

John, I. (1998). The scientist-practitioner model: A critical examination. *Australian Psychologist 33:* 24-30.

Kagan, C. and Lewis, S. (1990). Transforming psychological practice. *Australian Psychologist 25:* 270-280.

Kitzinger, C. (1991). Feminism, psychology and the paradox of power. *Feminism and Psychology 1:* 111-129.

Lapsley, H. and Wilkinson, S. (2001). Organizing feminist psychology in New Zealand. *Feminism and Psychology 11:* 386-392.

Levinson, D., Darrow, C., Klein, E., Levinson, M., and McKee, B. (1978). *The Seasons of a Man's Life.* New York: Knopf.

Marchant, H. and Wearing, B. (Eds.) (1986). *Gender Reclaimed: Women in Social Work.* Sydney: Hale and Ironmonger.

McCormick, T. (1991). "An analysis of some pitfalls of traditional mentoring for minorities and women in higher education." Paper presented at the Annual Meeting of the American Educational Research Association, April, Chicago, IL.

McWhirter, E. (1998). An empowerment model of counselor education. *Canadian Journal of Counseling/Revue Canadienne de Counseling 32*(1): 12-26.

Nelson, M. and Holloway, E. (1990). Relation of gender to power and involvement in supervision. *Journal of Counseling Psychology 37:* 473-479.

Payne, W.H. (1873). *School Supervision.* New York: American Book.

Perkins, R. (1991). Women with long-term mental health problems: Issues of power and powerlessness. *Feminism and Psychology 1:* 131-139.

Sherman, P. (1984). The counselor as change agent: A revolution? Not likely. *The Counselling Psychologist 12:* 111-116.

Shopland, J. (2000). Women and counseling: A feminist perspective. *Health-sharing Women 11*(2): 7-11.

Slack, P. J. F. (1990). "Power of the mind's eye." Paper presented at the Annual Meeting of the American Educational Research Association, April, Boston, MA.

Squire, C. (1990). Feminism as antipsychology: Learning and teaching in feminist psychology. In E. Burman (Ed.), *Feminists and Psychological Practice* (pp. 76-88). London: Sage.

Travers, C. (1986). "Feminist supervision: questions and answers." Unpublished paper, Palmerston North, NZ.

FURTHER READING

Hawkins, P. and Shohet, R. (2000). *Supervision in the Helping Professions* (Second Edition). Buckingham, UK: Open University Press.

Kitzinger, C. (1991). Feminism, psychology and the paradox of power. *Feminism and Psychology 1:* 111-129.

Nelson, M. and Holloway, E. (1990). Relation of gender to power and involvement in supervision. *Journal of Counseling Psychology 37:* 473-479.

Shopland, J. (2000). Women and counseling: A feminist perspective. *Health-sharing Women 11*(2): 7-11.

Chapter 15

Respectful Super-Vision:
Avoiding Relational Violence

Robert Doan

In this chapter Robert Doan invites us to consider the types of conversations between supervisors and trainees in therapy that are respectful and avoid relational violence. In an experiential didactic style he invites the reader to participate in the process of helpful supervision by addressing questions as if he or she were attending one of his seminars. Lists are generated contrasting descriptions of supervisors considered by trainees as "most helpful," as opposed to "psychonoxious" or violent in the relational sense of imposing their knowledge from above. No surprise that, for trainees, respectful supervision is relationally sensitive and collaborative in approach rather than highly directive and theory or model driven.

Here Doan contrasts Maturana's definition of *violence* as "holding an opinion to be true and demanding that others hold it as well" with *love,* which is "making space for someone to be near you." He includes a highly useful computer-based exercise for generating adjectives around current and preferred supervisory styles, which the reader can adapt to his or her own practice. The chapter concludes with further questions about the influence of supervision models on practice and suggests guidelines for a collaborative, relationally violence-free approach in the field.

Super: very large or powerful; great, excessive, above, in addition . . . higher in quality or degree or intensity . . . more than . . . in excessive degree or intensity . . . surpassing all or most others of its kind . . . situated or placed above . . . superior in title, status, or position.

Vision: something seen in a dream, trance, or fantasy . . . an object of imagination . . . a supernatural appearance that conveys a revelation . . . the act or power of imagination . . . unusual discernment or foresight . . . a mode of seeing or conceiving . . . a lovely or charming sight . . . direct mystical awareness of the supernatural.

Supervision: the action, process, or occupation of supervising . . . a critical watching and directing (as of activities or a course of action).

DECONSTRUCTING SUPER-VISION

In keeping with the postmodern and narrative tradition of deconstruction, this chapter begins with just such a process. The meanings attributed to "super-vision" in *Webster's* dictionary (1967) previously stated present a daunting challenge to anyone involved in this process. Indeed, even a cursory examination implies that a supervisor should possess an advanced and elite form of perception and conceiving. Upon deeper contemplation, the standard meaning of the two words combined suggests an even more privileged "vision"; one that might come from a *super*natural or spiritual origin . . . or, at the very least, an advanced form of intuition or accomplishment. That is, any *super*visor worth his or her salt will possess an insight and knowledge that is *super*ior to those being *super*vised. This implies a hierarchy of knowledge that situates the supervisor "above," and those being supervised "below," with the supervisor knowing something special which those in training do not have access to and thus must receive in some manner from the one with the privileged vision. Following this thinking, the supervisor's job can be conceptualized as correcting, editing, or somehow altering someone who is deficient or lacking into a *super*ior product via the imparting of special knowledge or techniques. It is not too far afield to suggest that most supervision is based on such assumptions, with little or no thought concerning the accuracy, effectiveness, or origins of these notions. That this has occurred via a slow-but-sure social process which "reified" such meanings (the process by a which a concept becomes accepted by a large group of people, or culture, as truth or reality *without* those involved in the process being aware that they have done so).

This can be further punctuated by the very clear and concise writings of Harlene Anderson (1997):

From this perspective the knower [supervisor] is autonomous and separate from that which he or she observes, describes, and explains, whether of a physical nature like a storm or of a human nature like crowd behavior. The individual knower is the source of and validator of all knowledge. The individual is privileged. (p. 30)

Thus, supervisors meet with their trainees, assume they possess some superior form of knowledge, and spend little or no time challenging the validity of this assumption. The intent of this chapter is to do just that; to "step back" from the traditional view of supervision, ask questions and ponder alternate conceptualizations, and invite the reader along for the ride . . . hopefully an enjoyable and informative one. The ride begins with a series of experiential exercises and concludes with a discussion of the implications. This is done in an attempt to simulate the type of conversational dialogues the author encourages when conducting classes and seminars on supervision. It is doubtful such a process can be duplicated in this format, but hopefully it will be superior to a one-sided monologue.

OUR SUPERVISION HISTORY/HERSTORY: DOES IT HAVE ANYTHING TO TEACH US?

When interacting with groups interested in improving their supervisory skills, I generally start by asking a series of questions and inviting their answers and discussion:

1. Do you want the supervision you provide to other therapists to be experienced by them as helpful? How important is it that this be the case?
2. Do you think that most therapists look forward to supervision sessions or dread them?
3. When you think back on all the supervision you have received as a therapist, how would you describe the instances you found most helpful? How would you describe the instances you found least helpful?

Prior to reading further, it is recommended that the reader carefully answer these questions. On number three it is suggested they make a list of the descriptors—helpful ones on one side of a page and not helpful ones on the other.

Most groups answer the questions in similar fashion, although there are, of course, individual differences. Question one is a "no brainer"; everyone shares the desire that his or her supervision be experienced as helpful by others.

What sense would the reader make of someone who is *not* interested in being helpful? What advice would you have for them?

Since most supervisors do desire to be helpful, some very important questions can be asked in relation to what "is" helpful. Are some types of helping efforts experienced as more helpful than others? Put simply, how is "being helpful" defined behaviorally? Is help detecting and pointing out that which is wrong and in need of correction? Or is it building upon strengths? Is help assuming that the trainee should "be like you"? Is what is helpful more likely to be defined by the supervisor or the one receiving the supervision? If the one being supervised is not experiencing the supervision as helpful, how important is this information to the supervisor?

I am reminded of something that Evan Imber-Black (1988; Imber-Black, Roberts, and Whiting, 1989), who was then director of training at the Family Therapy Program in Calgary, Canada, asked me during my doctoral internship. She wondered whether I wanted my help to actually be helpful to clients. I responded that I certainly did. She smiled and instructed me that all helping efforts are not created equal; that we should take special care to ensure what we are offering as help is actually being experienced as such by the client. I would offer this as equally valid in relation to the "help" we offer in the name of supervision.

Question two (do people look forward to supervision?) elicits more varied responses, but the "consensus" picture suggests that most people dread supervision for fear they will be found deficient, although most agree it depends entirely on the supervisor.

That brings us to the answers on question three (describe the best and worst supervision you're received). The following table is presented as a representative sample (Table 15.1).

TABLE 15.1. Characteristics of Best and Worst Supervisors

Supervisors who were most helpful	Supervisors who were "psychonoxious"
Understanding	All knowing
Warm	Detached
Empathetic	Insensitive
Nonjudgmental	Focused on "rules"
Full of ideas	Imposing ideas
Caring	Cold
Honest	Not trustworthy
Supervisee was first priority during session	Used session to discuss own issues
Secure, not easily threatened	Insecure, uneasy
Facilitative, not directive	Highly directive
Not fearful or anxious	Anxious
Love based	Fear based
Available	Hard to contact
Fair	Rule oriented
People based	Model or theory based

How did your list compare with the one in Table 15.1? Are there significant deletions or additions? (Feel free to share these with the author via e-mail at <rdoan@ucok.edu>. The more voices, the more complete the picture.)

Each time I experience such a conversation, I recall Humberto Maturana's definitions of love and violence shared during a workshop I was privileged to attend. Love was described as "making space for someone to be near you." He added that as rules increase, love decreases. Violence was defined as "holding an opinion to be true and demanding that others hold it as well," with physical attack being an extreme, but not the only form of such a demand.

In relation to these definitions, is it possible for supervision to be "violent"? Have you ever experienced such violence personally? What effect did it have on your life as a therapist and as a person? Did it invite you to be a better therapist? What *did* it invite you to do?

What sense do you make of "love is making space for someone to be near you"? Do you agree? Why would Maturana believe that rules decrease love? Think of the people you call your best friends. How much space is there for you to be near them? What creates such "space"?

Consider people you would rather not be around. How much space is there for you to be you? What lets you know there is no "space"?

PREFERRED VERSUS NONPREFERRED SUPERVISOR ADJECTIVES

At the University of Central Oklahoma, where I teach, we have developed a computer program called I-SPI, which allows us to catch a glimpse of people in the act of "psyching" (creating worlds via the stories and meanings they tell themselves). I include this instrument here in an abbreviated form for your interest and enjoyment (Figure 15.1).

Compare your two adjective "sorts." What adjectives were picked as very similar to your preferred supervisory style that were not picked as early in your current style? What type of characteristics would you like to increase? Have less of? What currently restrains you from "being" the supervisor you prefer to be?

You could, of course, do exactly the same process for "What is a helpful supervisor like?" and "What is a nonhelpful supervisor like?"

MORE QUESTIONS TO CONSIDER

The following questions are borrowed from Freedman and Combs (1996) and have been revised to render them relevant to supervision. In the original form they address the therapist's relationship with a client. Is our relationship with other therapists any less important?

1. How does the model/theory/style that you use to supervise invite you to "see" those that you are supervising?
2. How does it instruct you to conduct yourself during the supervision session?
3. How does it invite those being supervised to conduct themselves with you?
4. How does it have them "treat" themselves?

5. How are those you supervise being redefined or redescribed by what you do?
6. Does it invite supervisees to view the supervisor or themselves as being an expert on themselves?
7. Does it invite and isolate those being supervised or give them a sense of collaboration?
8. Is the supervision moving toward generative or normative results?
9. Does the model require that those being supervised enter the supervisor's knowledge and language, or does it require the supervisor to enter theirs?

What was your experience of reading and thinking about these questions? Did they invite comfort or discomfort? Why? Do you agree or disagree that supervisors should monitor their own behavior in such a manner?

WHAT DOES ALL THIS MEAN?

While I was in Calgary, completing the internship I mentioned previously, I was told a story by one of my fellow trainees. It was a story I could scarcely believe because it was so at odds with my perception of her as a therapist. She related that in a previous training venue, a supervisor told her that she was not suited to working as a therapist and should make a living in some other endeavor. She went on to say that only her acceptance into our current program had engendered enough hope for her to continue to believe she could be a good therapist.

I cite this as an example of relational violence, and while I do not claim to know anything concerning the intentions or perceptions of the previous supervisor, I will go so far as to say that a very gifted therapist was almost lost to the field. This would have been sad indeed.

Supervisors have a certain "gatekeeping" responsibility to ensure that therapists under their supervision do not perpetrate relational violence on the general public. In my perspective, this is a responsibility that goes with the territory of being a supervisor and is an important component indeed. However, unless we are very careful, we may

Adjective List

Worrying	Good Natured	Careful	Nervous
Persevering	Clownish	Sociable	Interested
Forgiving	Original	Acquiescent	Insecure
Affectionate	Average	Talkative	Daring
	Reliable	Unemotional	

Referring to this list of adjectives, fill in the following chart by asking yourself the question: *What is my current supervisory style like?* (Use an adjective only once; pick one very similar, then one very dissimilar, two similar, two dissimilar, etc.)

                  ____

                  ____

                  ____

       ____   ____   ____

   ____ ____ ____ ____ ____

____ ____ ____ ____ ____ ____ ____

very	a lot	little	some	little	a lot	very
much						much

Dissimilar   Similar

———→ Work from extremes to the center ←———

Do the procedure again, only this time ask yourself the question, *What is my preferred supervisory style like?*

                  ____

                  ____

                  ____

       ____   ____   ____

   ____ ____ ____ ____ ____

____ ____ ____ ____ ____ ____ ____

very	a lot	little	some	little	a lot	very
much						much

Dissimilar   Similar

———→ Work from extremes to the center ←———

FIGURE 15.1. I-SPI Instrument

unwittingly become perpetrators ourselves. And more, we can do so "righteously" in the name of the truth of a particular model, theory, or philosophy. We can do so in the process of trying to make "clones" of those we supervise, or in the reluctance to take a critical look at our "sacred" beliefs. Indeed, this would be very likely if we fall under the influence of the traditional meaning of *super*-vision and the expert and entitled stance it invites.

So, how can we uphold our gatekeeping responsibility and be as nonviolent as possible? The last portion of this chapter will address this question by offering suggestions that are based upon the previous exercises and questions.

1. *Stay aware that everything is subject to interpretation.* Much depends on who you believe you are and what you believe you are trying to do. Motives are extremely important, objectives highly influence outcomes, and life proceeds forth from our intentions. We must first be aware enough to be very clear about this with ourselves. Are we more interested in our help being helpful or in being "right"? What motives and intentions do we bring to the supervision session? Are we teachers? Are we moral enforcers? Are we friendly co-collaborators? Is there actually room for what is helpful to be worked out "between" the supervisor and supervisee instead of being known ahead of time by the supervisor? Can supervisory conversations be viewed as explorations of various interpretations and the implications for conducting therapy? The following questions are offered as examples of the intention to coconstruct what is helpful with those we supervise:

- What would you like to address in the time we have together? Are there particular aspects of the counseling process you would like to concentrate on?
- What sort of responses would you like from me? Would you prefer direct advice, questions, reflections, or a mix of these? What do you think/feel would be most helpful for you?
- What are your personal goals as a counselor at present? Are there particular things you are working on that you would like me to listen or watch for in the session?

- Which model or theory of therapy informs your work? Do you want me to supervise you to the best of my ability from this model, or introduce ideas from other frames?
- It is my wish and intent that these sessions be helpful to you. Can you let me know if they are not? Can we have that sort of agreement?

2. *How the message is given is more important than how it is received.* I am again reminded of a conversation I had with Evan Imber-Black during my internship. She commented that in a session held earlier that day, that I had "opened many doors that I was too polite to walk through." I can remember being struck by how kindly she had just told me to "follow up" on some of my lines of inquiry. She suggested that my reluctance to hurt or embarrass people might be stopping me from having the type of detailed conversations that would be helpful, and inquired whether I thought that might be the case. (I did think so.)

There are many ways to deliver supervisory messages. These can vary widely in the extent to which they are received as being helpful. In general, those that positively connote the behavior of the supervisee, will stand a greater chance of being heard without defensiveness or hurt. A "default" which is suggested here, is that we give those we supervise the benefit of the doubt, in other words, they are doing what they are doing with some positive intention. In short, they are trying to help.

3. *Be aware that we are "in relationship" with those we supervise.* What follows is borrowed from the writings of Harlene Anderson (1997). I have altered her words slightly to make them more relevant to the topic of supervision.

> What is implied is the need for a consistent, ongoing analysis of our supervisory traditions; of the way we are in relationship with the people we supervise, of the way we think, talk, act with, and are responsive to them. This invites us to pause and reflect, to daily be aware enough to "deconstruct" our interactions with those we supervise, and assess and evaluate these interactions regularly.

My interpretation of her words suggests that we need to be individually aware and responsible for the supervision that we offer, and that the relationship we have with those we supervise is the most important variable. It is far more important than any theory, model, or domain of knowledge.

4. *Call what we do "collaboration" instead of supervision.* Perhaps it is time for a "languaging" change? Is it possible that the meanings that have socially evolved in relation to "supervisor" have outlived their usefulness? If we called what we do "super-collaboration" how would it change our thoughts, feelings, and behaviors? This is a vivid example of being clear about who we are and what we are trying to do. As I have considered this perspective, it has led to the following ways of "being" with those I "supervise":

- Asking the therapist what he or she wants me to watch or listen for in the session under review.
- Suggesting that therapists review tapes of their own work and first pick out everything they did or said that they want to continue doing and saying with clients (instead of picking out that which is "wrong").
- Using teams that offer reflections to therapists in much the same way they do with clients.
- Conducting personal interviews that call forth a clear picture of the therapist the trainee wants to be, in other words, their preferred therapist narrative.
- Conducting personal interviews that explore the particular personal gifts that the therapist feels can serve him or her well in doing therapy.
- Providing trainees with the opportunity to serve on reflecting teams as often as possible.

5. *Judgment and guilt paralyze while awareness and love mobilize.* Seek to establish an atmosphere in the supervision/collaboration context that is as free of fear and judgment as possible. All of us know how paralyzing it is to be afraid of judgment and reprisal, and we have all experienced the liberation of love and acceptance. It might be well to consider the important differences between the two, and conduct our supervisory sessions accordingly. What more needs to be said?

CONCLUDING REMARKS

Collaborative, violence-free supervision is difficult to achieve if one falls under the influence of traditional, modernist, bedrock assumptions. Most of us have been raised in cultures that reified such assumptions to the extent that they became "truth," which led to certain notions concerning the form that "help" should take. It requires much awareness, practice, and intention to escape the influence of this "grand narrative" and alter our supervisory styles. It is hoped that this chapter has provided a springboard for thinking about supervision in ways that will yield more satisfying supervisory experiences for both the supervisor and supervisee.

REFERENCES

Anderson, H. (1997). *Conversation, Language, and Possibilities*. New York: Basic Books.

Freedman, J. and Combs, G. (1996). *Narrative Therapy: The Social Construction of Preferred Realities*. New York: W.W. Norton and Co.

Imber-Black, E. (1988). *Families and Larger Systems: A Therapist's Guide Through the Labyrinth*. New York: Guilford Press.

Imber-Black, E., Roberts, J., and Whiting, R. (1989). *Rituals in Families and Family Therapy*. New York: W. W. Norton and Co.

Webster's Seventh New Collegiate Dictionary (1967). Chicago, IL: Rand-McNally.

SUGGESTED READINGS

Doan, R. and Clifton, D. (1990). The reauthoring of therapist's stories. *Journal of Strategic and Systemic Therapies* 9(4): 61-66.

Freedman, J. and Combs, G. (1996). *Narrative Therapy: The Social Construction of Preferred Realities*. New York: W.W. Norton and Co.

Parry, A. and Doan, R. (1994). *Story Re-Visions: Narrative Therapy in the Post-Modern World*. New York: Guilford Press.

White, M. (1990). Family therapy training and supervision in a world of experience and narrative. In White, M. and Epston, D. *Experience, Contradiction, Narrative, and Experience* (pp. 75-95). Adelaide, Australia: Dulwich Centre Publications.

Zimmerman, Z. and Dickerson, V. (1996). *If Problems Talked: Narrative Therapy in Action*. New York: Guilford Press.

*RESEARCH:
EXPLORING FROM WITHIN—
COLLABORATIVE RESEARCH
PRACTICES*

Chapter 16

Meaningful Moments As Collaborative Accomplishments: Research from Within Consultative Dialogue

Tom Strong

Most often, research data are characterized as a commodity that one "gets" from willing participants. When that process of procurement is enacted with sufficient "rigor," it is assumed that what the researcher walks away with is close to the "reality" of what the participant experienced. This description (among other limitations) fails to capture the ways in which the researcher's contribution is integral to the participant's experience—how the very act of asking a question brings interviewer and interviewee to new understandings that they fashion together, through dialogue. In this sense, research is not simply an act of *finding out,* but is also always a *creating together* process. In this chapter, Tom Strong brings a finely attuned sensitivity to the dynamics of discourse to a qualitative research process. The launching point is a question about what clients find "meaningful" in therapy; but rather than taking the opportunity to purportedly learn what therapeutic experiences contribute to meaningful moments, Strong examines the impact of the question itself. The goal of this process is not to seek conclusions about counseling process, but rather to further a conversation devoted to a question about meaningfulness, and the experience it generates.

I know I am a fool, trying to make connections out of scraps but how else is there to proceed? The fragmentariness of life makes coherence suspect but to babble is a different kind of treachery. Perhaps it is a vanity. Am I vain enough to assume you will understand me? No. So I go on puzzling over new joints for words, hoping that this time, one piece will slide smooth against the next . . . Walk with me.

Jeannette Winterson, 1997, p. 24

How do conversations "give birth" to meanings? This question tugs at my curiosity, given my discursive orientation (e.g., Edwards, 1997; Gergen, 1999; Potter, 1996) to practice as a therapist and therapy researcher. Thinking discursively as a practitioner-researcher, I believe that I am involved in a poetic process in which "respondents" are as active in their meaning-making efforts as I am.

Most therapy research is conducted on, for, about, and (sometimes) with participants in therapy. Most research suggests therapy is administered to clients, to be assessed for its effect—as if clients were inert and therapists supplied active ingredients to move them "therapeutically" (Bohart, O'Hara, and Leitner, 1998). Although increasing emphasis is being given to collaborative qualitative research on therapy (Hill, Thompson, and Nutt-Williams, 1997), few take up John Shotter's (1984, 1993, 1995) challenge to see meaning-making activities (such as those in therapy) as taking place in "joint action," *within* relationships.

RESEARCH AS CONVERSATION

In connected knowing one enters into stories beyond the bounds of one's experience.

Blythe McVicker-Clinchy, 1996, p. 238

Some qualitative researchers see research as conversation (Kvale, 1996; Scheurich, 1995). Alternately, therapy has been characterized as collaborative research (Andersen, 1997). How, then, should we regard claims that questions asked by research assistants were regarded by respondents as more therapeutic than those asked in therapy (Gale, Odell, and Nagireddy, 1995)? Whether intended or not, our questions can be invitations into a collaborative research process of meaning making. How we regard our role in such a process, ethically and pragmatically, has implications for its potentials.

Many feel a difference in their bodies when on a forensic quest for fact, as opposed to when they elicit accounts or opinions from people. Forensic conversation is about "getting things right," while other forms of conversation welcome subjectivity. "Getting things right" seems an onerous task, premised on the idea that conversation can yield certainty. Qualitative research generally eschews "rhetoric of discovery or revelation" (Burman, 1997) because we constructionists cannot, as traditional researchers claim, "use talk to construct a sense of a talk-independent reality" (Sampson, 1993, p. 180).

Having been influenced by dialogue theorists (Bakhtin, 1981; Morson and Emerson, 1990), I approach research conversations with new concerns. Do they have a role-bound, asymmetric tilt where the researcher has greater influence over the content and process of the conversation (Drew, 1991)? Steier (1991) calls research participants "our reciprocators," highlighting the interdependence between researchers and "subjects." Traditional therapy research sanctions conversations to be under the control of the researcher (Heron, 1996).

Inescapably, we all participate in "life's gigantic conversation" (Newman and Holzman, 1997), in webs of conversation beyond, but related to, research conversations. Indeed, any claims of "knowing" seem to only further conversation, instead of bringing (as in the purported case of scientific objectivity) closure or convergence (Billig, 1996). Just when the ideas of Newton appeared to have cornered the possibilities of natural science, along came the ideas of Einstein.

RESEARCH AND THE IMMEDIACIES
OF CONVERSATION

Proximity is beyond intentionality.

Zygmunt Bauman, 1993, p. 87

Bauman's admonition implies our intentions alone cannot determine how our talking with others will go. There is no self to bracket off in research conversations. We inescapably influence, and are influenced by, our conversational partners (Strong, 2000). Where we go from this understanding concerns me. Much research is undertaken with a sense that we can *de-relate*—to some extent—from our research partners, to go outside our relationship to comment on its products and proceedings like a stranger. For Bauman, relational proximity, and the immediacies of conversation, blows that pipedream for us.

Although research *on* psychotherapy is still conducted in lab settings using controlled procedures with discrete variables, this is a practice Kazdin considers "well intentioned but oversimplified" (1994,

p. 66). Recently many quantitative and qualitative methods for studying therapy processes and outcomes have been developed (McLeod, 1999). Within qualitative research, one can now read accounts of therapy derived from ethnographic (Smith, Sells, and Clevenger, 1994); feminist (Myers-Avis and Turner, 1995); grounded theory (Watson and Rennie, 1994); discourse analytic (Kogan and Brown, 1998); conversation analytic (Gale, 1992); narrative analytic (Holstein and Gubrium, 2000); phenomenological (Boss, Dahl, and Kaplan, 1995); and hermeneutic (Walsh, Perrucci, and Severns, 1999) methods. For the most part (exception: Myers-Avis and Turner, 1995), these advances, while adding nuanced understandings of the therapy experience, come from research *on* therapy. Steve de Shazer (1994) suggests that conversations cannot help us get down to the bottom of things; instead, their meanings are simultaneously shaped by *and* shaping of the conversations in which they take place (Heritage, 1984).

Kvale (1996), contrasts miner (bedrock truth can be found) and traveler (wandering together in conversation) metaphors in qualitative research. Much therapy research seeks knowledge to intervene correctly (miner metaphor), assuming knowledge from particular contexts applies to all. This "scientist-practitioner" orientation requires the distance, neutral (?) morals, and a ratio-technical relationship to clients and their problems found in our codes of ethics (example: American Association for Marriage and Family Therapy, 1991). But this encourages disengagement from the very conversations therapists participate in as coconstructors of change. It is difficult to be "scientifically" part of an engaging therapy conversation, so I have sought ethical and accountable ideas—focused on the mutualities of meaning making—to inform my research (Ellis, Kiesinger, and Tillman-Healy, 1997; Grafanaki, 1996).

CONVERSATION AND THE YET-TO-BE-SPOKEN

Reclaiming a voice . . . has also been about reclaiming, reconnecting and reordering those ways of knowing which were submerged, hidden or driven underground.

Linda Tuhiwai Smith, 1999, p. 69

Discursive approaches to research ask us to accept our participation in the yet-to-be-spoken. For a discursive researcher there is no re-telling of stories, only tellings, since each telling is uniquely influenced by temporal, social, and other circumstances (Holstein and Gubrium, 2000). How does my participation in conversations of inquiry shape what I am told? What happens when asking clients to make distinctions in previously unarticulated areas of their lives?

I seek methods that position the researcher as a coresearcher *with* clients, as someone contributing to the processes and outcomes of therapy we want to better understand. This approximates Donald Schon's (1983) reflective practitioner, someone responsive in bringing theory and evolving circumstance together when interacting with clients. However, most studies de-emphasize the immediacies of interaction in therapy—where I contend that we do our best work. Missing is a view of our questions as *performative;* in that they can evoke, construct, and even invite positions on and experiences from which generative dialogues can emerge. "Performative" is a way of characterizing the improvisational activities involved in dialogues and social interaction. Humans are regarded as interactionally creative and responsive to one another in ways that go beyond scripted, or cause-effect relations.

CONVERSATIONAL RESEARCH FROM WITHIN

All our talk— whether about 'things' as such, or our more poetic talk that creates new possibilities between us—is simply rooted or grounded in our interwoven ways of relational talking and acting, and . . . in nothing more!

John Shotter, 1994, p. 7

My preferred research picture draws from John Shotter, who has been inspired by dialogue theorist Mikhail Bakhtin (1981; Morson and Emerson, 1990), philosopher Ludwig Wittgenstein, and Russian developmental psychologist, Lev Vygotsky. Shotter (1984) sees "joint action" involved in creating meanings and coordinating practices from *within* relationships. We cannot just say anything because sensitivities, relational traditions, and contexts are involved in coordinating how we communicate with one anther. Our conversations are like meetings of microcultures (Strong, 2002) where we work out how we will talk, and about what. Much occurs aside from making utterances and hearing them that helps us accomplish what we do when communicating in our relationships. Though conversation analysts (Hutchby and Wooffitt, 1998) and ethnomethodologists (Heritage, 1984) have examined communicative practices that create social orders in which these accomplishments take place, these methods still place them external to the orders they attempt to explain. Shotter's (1984, 1993, 1999; Shotter and Katz, 1999) work begs us to step inside, to see what comes from our participation in conversations. Specifically, my primary interest relates to how "new" meanings and conversational practices are developed in therapy. I share Harlene Anderson's (1997) view that therapy helps when it makes preferred differences in *how* clients talk to others, including themselves.

VARIATIONS ON A POETIC METHOD

To the cry "back to the things . . . themselves," I answer, "back further—not to the things, but to our descriptions that construct whatever we are looking at as things."

Robert Russell, 1994, p. 182

I am curious about how clients answer: what happens in therapeutic conversation, in moments they regard as "meaningful"? I am interested in the "whats" and the "hows" of conversation's interplay offered in their answers. While wary of lifting conversational shards out of the flow of interaction that created them, the research I highlight focuses on multiple meanings and meaning-making possibilities accomplishable in the course of conversation. This research borrows from "social poetics," a view of meaning-making articulated by John Shotter and Arlene Katz (1999; Katz and Shotter, 1996).

Recently, Margaret Fuller completed a thesis (Fuller, 2000; Fuller and Strong, 2001) with me focusing on meaningful moments identified by clients, especially given what took place when discussing these with them. She used interpersonal process recall (IPR) (Kagan, 1975), a method in which clients select videotaped moments from their ongoing therapy to later discuss with her—in this case, a moment that felt "most alive" to them. Where her study differed from others using IPR was that she saw her "research" as constructive. This move fits with comments from IPR researcher David Rennie (2000), who questioned the discovery-like (miner metaphor) claims made from this kind of research. Margaret saw herself actively contributing to her research outcomes, much like traditional action researchers, except from *within* her research/therapy relationships. She was interested in what occurs when she invited people to revisit meaningful moments, for the meaningful possibilities and pathways of conversation they might generate.

Late in her interviews Margaret asked: did her coresearchers see their "alive moments" as spiritual in any way? She hoped they would respond by speaking from within this different discourse (a spiritual one) as if it was an invitation they could take up or decline. She transcribed the poetic process they worked out between them in generatively speaking using this particularized form of discourse in therapy. Margaret's research highlighted several conversational developments as she and her coresearchers together considered, then took up, her invitation. Each person, for example, requested a definition of "spirituality"; and in hearing Margaret's open-ended definition moved to very tentative utterances ("well it's kind of like this . . ."), which they codeveloped into a fuller "spiritual account" that satisfied each coresearcher. Checking back three months after the initial interviews, each coresearcher reported having independently devoted further consideration to the role of "spirituality" in their lives. Margaret's research exemplified how coconstructing sensitive and significant meaning can occur in discursive approaches to therapy, something I will not have space to explain further here (Fuller, 2000; Fuller and Strong, 2001).

Margaret's research was part of a larger program of research of interest to me. Specifically, I seek research that illustrates the infinite poetic possibilities through which client-preferred meanings are created in therapy. Focusing up close, this research regards each conversational turn as a possible site for creating preferred meaning (Strong, 2002), though the regularities of conversation have a seamless quality that lull us into overlooking meaningful possibilities.

> The perceiving process becomes routinized by language. Its active participation sleep-walks inside the clothing of linguistic categories. Then people do not really pay heed to what is going on in the perceiving process. (Heron, 1996, p. 116)

These "sites" of routine and regularity (where "reality" is maintained through conversation—Berger and Luckmann, 1967) offer entry points to new discourses or "language games" (Wittgenstein, 1958), as possibly more generative ways to talk. Such entry points are where "Human beings (can) become who we 'are' by . . . being who we 'aren't' " (Newman and Holzman, 1997, p. 110).

Such inquiry in therapy is consistent with that of Norwegian psychiatrist Tom Andersen (1991), the originator of reflecting teams. His emphasis on multiple conversational possibilities when responding to clients—from which they can choose those most fitting their preferences and circumstances—is now widely adopted by "postmodern" therapists (e.g., Friedman, 1995). My research, and the therapies it emulates, aims to engage clients in new forms of conversation so as to coconstruct meanings they consider useful. Its point is not to discover generalizations about the therapy process, but to exemplify the possibilities gained by using a discursive approach to meaning making in therapy.

In terms of a "method," I offer the following orienting ideas:

1. Consider each conversational turn a site where contributions (those of you and your coresearchers) uphold or consolidate existing meanings and discourses. Conversely, consider each turn a possible prompt to converse in unfamiliar and generative ways.
2. Structure, or look for, opportunities to follow what happens together when inviting or shifting to other (ideally, useful and more generative) discourses.
3. Notice how your participation, your coresearchers', and your mutual participation, tentatively codevelops new meanings and ways of talking, especially if beginning to speak from an unaccustomed but invited discourse.
4. Notice the "dialogic dance" you develop as you find synchrony in your new ways of talking, or keep the conversation going so as to find a "shared dance step."
5. Notice what you do to keep things feeling mutual (and observe closely) when trying on new ways of talking, noticing when you are "stepping on the toes" of your conversational partner. Regard these as improvisational moves, not generally applicable conversational practices.

6. If you, like Margaret, want to explore the effect of a specific conversational invitation, you can try this using specific conversational practices from different therapies (examples: externalization or deconstructive questions) as invitations to new forms of talking.

Many possibilities come up for me in thinking this way about meaning making in therapy. What are the conversational back and forths that result when adopting new forms of therapeutic conversation? How are these backs and forths related to the meanings generated from them? How do people access "new" conversational resources (McNamee and Gergen, 1999) in these backs and forths, and how does the use of these resources evoke others relevant to the relationship? How do clients and therapists "cosignify" meaningful moments, those they select as sites for shifting to alternative forms of talking? What conversational practices do we bring to such interactions that are perceived as generative to clients or research participants? How do participants identify moments "pregnant with" or "bereft of" meaningful possibilities? These are a few of the curiosities I hold regarding the potentials involved in this way of conceptualizing therapy research.

SOME ETHICAL CAVEATS

When someone reflects-in-action, he becomes a researcher in the practice context. He is not dependent on the categories of established theory and technique, but . . . does not separate thinking from doing, ratiocinating his way to a decision which he must later convert to action. Because his experimenting is a kind of action, implementation is built into his inquiry.

Donald Schon, 1983, p. 69

Many feel ethically queasy about this approach to research, especially if they are unfamiliar with the improvisationally-styled practices of the discursive therapies. Missing from Schon's words is a conversational *other* with whom all this reflexive improvising must occur. Fully "collaborative" relationships can promote a slippery slope toward an abuse of power, blurring the boundary between a traditional researcher and the subject of her or his research (Grafanaki, 1996).

This was a matter of intense discussion: if Margaret's research had the power to influence others, how could she interact in ethically constructive ways (Strong, 2000)? This research is interventive, requiring sensitivities to avoid dominating the meanings and ways of talk created between clients and researchers/therapists (Weingarten, 1991), as well as transcribing and interpreting meanings from their conversations (Alcoff, 1991). Just as a moment can be given new meanings by speaking anew to it, so this can happen in transcribing or revisiting transcribed meanings. This raises the ethical question of how such conversations can collaboratively be ended, should they seem continually generative of meaningful possibilities. The answer needs to come from within the relationship, when, together with our co-researchers, we decide to call it quits because our conversation has gone far enough.

Those believing in only empirically validated research or clinical interventions (Henry, 1998) will feel particularly uncomfortable. Although semistructured interviews are used, with qualitative research software (N-Vivo, 1999) to organize the "data," no standardized protocol is necessary. Such standards are considered hegemonic and restrictive of the very generative possibilities under study (Russell, 1994). In John Shotter's words, "Embedded in our everyday activities—out in the world between us, not hidden behind appearances—are the methods we need" (1999, p. 11). The key here obviously rests with practicing in a manner regarded as accountable, or "relationally responsible" by our coresearchers (McNamee and Gergen, 1999). To optimize this relational responsibility, working as part of a consultative team, follow-ups with participants to ensure that their meanings were honored in the final write-up, and constantly interrogating one's own intentions and practices are suggested.

A final caveat rests with the value of such research to therapists and clients. This research seeks no generalizable results. It was undertaken to highlight the infinite conversational possibilities that result when flexibly and collaboratively elaborating on unvoiced experiences. In so doing, the challenge is to keep conversations and meanings fresh, and not bound to the routines of our institutional or cultural discourses as Kogan and Brown (1998) highlight:

> By continually assessing how we practice culture with others as a discursive activity, we hope to keep all such notions "in play" and resist the "sedimentation" of social facts that may later be understood to be sources of oppression. (p. 511)

Consistent with this view, social therapists Fred Newman and Lois Holzman (1997) caution us about "fetishizing and fossilizing" our meanings and practices in ways that alienate us from participating in life meaningfully. The research I propose invites participants into unfamiliar dialogues, to actively co-author new experiences. Participating this way together—how it unfolds and what it produces—is the focus here.

IMPLICATIONS

> The hermeneutic circle in daily life is everyone's everyday "research" (or speculating) model.

> Tom Andersen, 1997, p. 126

Some might wonder what the value of research that makes no claims of generalizable utility is. For me, this research and its "findings" hopefully prompts practitioners to reflect on their professional and institutional discourses (Drew and Sorjonen, 1997), for how these, and other aspects of our communications, can affect clients. I hope this spurs therapists on to greater flexibility and creativity in their work with clients. I am intrigued by the social poetics work of John Shotter and Arlene Katz (1999; Katz and Shotter, 1996), for what it suggests about how meanings are created in relationships. I want to explore what happens when people are invited to converse in unaccustomed, but generative, ways.

For John Shotter, "until recently we have ignored the part played in our lives by our living, dialogically-structured, responsive relations within our surroundings" (1999, p. 11). His concern is that conversations focus too much on the familiar (their meanings and practices), thereby obscuring opportunities when unrealized possibilities for preferred meaning and action could develop. The research I have been describing highlights socially poetic opportunities for the meaningful potentials they offer to coresearchers. It asks us to consider how we could optimize the meaning-making potentials those immanent opportunities afford while better attuning us to the effects our accustomed conversational practices play in bypassing such opportunities.

REFERENCES

Alcoff, L. (1991). The problem of speaking for others. *Cultural Critique* 20: 5-32.

American Association for Marriage and Family Therapy. (1991). *Code of Ethics.* Washington, DC: Author.

Andersen, T. (1991). *The reflecting team.* New York: Norton.

Andersen, T. (1997). Researching client-therapist relationships: A collaborative study for informing therapy. *Journal of Systemic Therapies* 16: 125-133.

Anderson, H. (1997). *Conversation, language and possibilities.* New York: Basic.

Bakhtin, M. (1981). *The dialogic imagination.* Austin: University of Texas Press.

Bauman, Z. (1993). *Postmodern ethics.* Oxford: Blackwell.

Berger, P. and Luckmann, T. (1967). *The social construction of reality.* New York: Anchor.

Billig, M. (1996). *Arguing and Thinking: A rhetorical approach to social psychology,* Second edition. Cambridge, UK: Cambridge University Press.

Bohart, A., O'Hara, M., and Leitner, L. (1998). Empirically violated treatments: Disenfranchisement of humanistic and other psychotherapies. *Psychotherapy Research* 8(2): 141-157.

Boss, P., Dahl, C. and Kaplan, L. (1995). The use of phenomenology in family therapy research: The search for meaning. In D. Sprenkle and S. Moon (Eds.), *Research methods in family therapy* (pp. 83-106). New York: Guilford.

Burman, E. (1997). Minding the gap: Positivism, psychology, and the politics of qualitative methods. *Journal of Social Issues* 53: 786-801.

de Shazer, S. (1994). *Words were originally magic.* New York: Norton.

Drew, P. (1991). Asymmetries of knowledge in conversational interactions. In I. Markova and K. Foppa (Eds.), *Asymmetries in dialogue* (pp. 21-48). Savage, MD: Barnes and Noble Books.

Drew, P. and Sorjonen, M. (1997). Institutional dialogue. In T. van Dijk (Ed.), *Discourse as social interaction,* Volume 2 (pp. 92-118). Thousand Oaks, CA: Sage.

Edwards, D. (1997). *Discourse and cognition.* London: Sage.

Ellis, C., Kiesinger, C., and Tillman-Healy, L. (1997). Interactive interviewing: Talking about emotional experience. In R. Hertz (Ed.), *Reflexivity and Voice* (pp. 119-149). Thousand Oaks, CA: Sage.

Friedman, S. (Ed.) (1995). *The reflecting team in action.* New York: Guilford.

Fuller, M. (2000). "Moments of "aliveness" in counseling: An untapped spiritual dimension?" Master of education thesis, University of Northern British Columbia.

Fuller, M. and Strong, T. (2001). Inviting passage to new discourse: "Alive moments" and their spiritual significance. *Counseling and Psychotherapy Research* 1(3): 200-214.

Gale, J. (1992). *Conversation analysis of therapeutic discourse: The pursuit of a therapeutic agenda.* Norwood, NJ: Ablex.

Gale, J., Odell, M., and Nagireddy, C. (1995). Marital therapy and self-reflexive research: Research and/as intervention. In G. Morris and R. Chenail (Eds.), *The talk of the clinic: Explorations in the analysis of medical and therapeutic discourse* (pp. 105-129). Hillsdale, NJ: Lawrence Erlbaum and Associates.

Gergen, K. (1999). *An invitation to social construction.* Thousand Oaks, CA: Sage.

Grafanaki, S. (1996). How research can change the researcher: The need for sensitivity, flexibility and ethical boundaries in conducting qualitative research in counseling/psychotherapy. *British Journal of Guidance and Counseling* 24: 329-338.

Henry, W. (1998). Science, politics, and the politics of science: The use and misuse of empirically validated treatment research. *Psychotherapy Research* 8: 126-140.

Heritage, J. (1984). *Garfinkel and ethnomethodology.* Cambridge, UK: Polity Press.

Heron, J. (1996). *Cooperative inquiry.* Thousand Oaks, CA: Sage.

Hill, C.E., Thompson, B.J., and Nutt-Williams, E. (1997). A guide to conducting consensual qualitative research. *Counseling Psychologist* 25: 517-572.

Holstein, J. and Gubrium, J. (2000). *The self we live by: Narrative identity in a postmodern world.* New York: Oxford Books.

Hutchby, I. and Wooffitt, R. (1998). *Conversation analysis: Principles, practices and applications.* Cambridge, UK: Polity Press.

Kagan, N. (1975). *Interpersonal process recall: A method for influencing human interaction.* (Available from N. Kagan, Educational Psychology Department, University Park, Houston, TX, 77004.)

Katz, A. and Shotter, J. (1996). Hearing the patient's "voice": Toward a social poetics in diagnostic interviews. *Social Science in Medicine* 43: 919-931.

Kazdin, A. (1994). Methodology, design and evaluation in psychotherapy research. In A. Bergin and S. Garfield (Eds.), *Handbook of psychotherapy and behavior change* (Fourth Edition) (pp. 19-71). New York: John Wiley and Sons.

Kogan, S. and Brown, A. (1998). Reading against the lines: Resisting foreclosure in therapy discourse. *Family Process* 37: 495-512.

Kvale, S. (1996). *InterViews.* Thousand Oaks, CA: Sage.

McLeod, J. (1999). *Practitioner research in counseling.* London: Sage.

McNamee, S. and Gergen, K. (Eds.) (1999). *Relational responsibility.* Thousand Oaks, CA: Sage.

McVicker Clinchy, B. (1996). Connected and separate knowing: Toward a marriage of two minds. In N. Rule Goldberger, J. Mattuck Tarule, B. McVicker Clinchy, and M. Field Belenky (Eds.), *Knowledge, difference, and power* (pp. 205-247). New York: Basic.

Morson, G. and Emerson, C. (1990). *Mikhail Bakhtin: Creation of a prosaics.* Stanford, CA: Stanford University Press.

Myers-Avis, J. and Turner, J. (1995). Feminist lenses in family therapy research: Gender, politics, and science. In D. Sprenkle and S. Moon (Eds.), *Research methods in family therapy* (pp. 145-169). New York: Guilford.

Newman, F. and Holzman, L. (1997). *The end of knowing.* New York: Routledge.

N-Vivo (1999). *NUD*IST Vivo software.* Melbourne, Australia: Qualitative Solutions and Research.

Potter, J. (1996). *Representing reality.* Thousand Oaks, CA: Sage.

Rennie, D. (2000). Aspects of the client's conscious control of the psychotherapeutic process. *Journal of Psychotherapy Integration* 10: 151-167.

Russell, R. (1994). Critically reading psychotherapy process research: A brief enactment. In R. Russell (Ed.), *Reassessing psychotherapy research* (pp. 166-184). New York: Guilford.

Sampson, E. (1993). *Celebrating the other.* Boulder, CO: Westview.

Scheurich, J. (1995). A postmodernist critique of research interviewing. *Qualitative Studies in Education* 8: 239-252.

Schon, D. (1983). *The reflective practitioner.* New York: Basic.

Shotter, J. (1984). *Social accountability and selfhood.* Oxford: Blackwell.

Shotter, J. (1993). *Conversational realities: Constructing life through language.* London: Sage.

Shotter, J. (1994). *Social constructionism and "providential dialogues."* An online paper available at <http://www.massey.ac.nz/~alock/virtual/provide.htm>.

Shotter, J. (1995). In conversation: Joint action, shared intentionality and ethics. *Theory and Psychology* 5: 49-73.

Shotter, J. (1999). *Dialogue, depth, and life inside responsive orders: From external observation to participatory understanding.* Online paper available at <http://pubpages.unh.edu/~jds/Performing_Knowledge.htm>.

Shotter, J. and Katz, A. (1999). "Living moments" in dialogic exchanges. *Human Systems* 9: 81-93.

Smith, T., Sells, S., and Clevenger, T. (1994). Ethnographic content analysis of couple and therapist perceptions in a reflecting team setting. *Journal of Marital and Family Therapy* 20: 267-286.

Steier, F. (1991). Reflexivity and methodology: An ecological constructionism. In F. Steier (Ed.), *Research and reflexivity* (pp. 163-185). Newbury Park, CA: Sage.

Strong, T. (2000). Collaborative influence. *Australian and New Zealand Journal of Family Therapy* 23: 144-148.

Strong, T. (2002). Dialogue in therapy's "borderzone." *Journal of Constructivist Psychology* 15: 245-262.

Tuhiwai Smith, L. (1999). *Decolonizing methodologies.* New York: Zed Books.

Walsh, R., Perrucci, A., and Severns, J. (1999). What's in a good moment: A hermeneutic study of psychotherapy values across levels of psychotherapeutic training. *Psychotherapy Research* 9: 304-326.

Watson, J. and Rennie, D. (1994). Qualitative analysis of clients' subjective experience of significant moments during exploration of problematic reactions. *Journal of Counseling Psychology* 41: 500-509.

Weingarten, J. (1991). The discourses of intimacy: Adding a social constructionist and feminist view. *Family Process* 30: 285-305.

Winterson, J. (1997). *Gut symmetries.* New York: Alfred Knopf.

Wittgenstein, L. (1958). *Philosophical investigations* (Third Edition) (G. Anscombe, Trans.) New York: Macmillan.

SUGGESTED READINGS

Fuller, M. and Strong, T. (2001). Inviting passage to new discourse: "Alive" moments and invitations to spiritual discourse. *Counseling and Psychotherapy Research* 1(3): 200-214.

Harre, R. and Langenhove, L. (Eds.) (1999). *Positioning theory: Moral contexts of intentional action.* Oxford: Blackwell.

McNamee, S. and Gergen, K. (Eds.) (1999). *Relational responsibility.* Thousand Oaks, CA: Sage.

Newman, F. and Holzman, L. (1997). *The end of knowing.* New York: Routledge.

Shotter, J. and Katz, A. (1999). "Living moments" in dialogic exchanges. *Human Systems* 9: 81-93.

Chapter 17

"Acting-With": Partisan Participant Observation As a Social-Practice Basis for Shared Knowing

Carla Willig
John Drury

Carla Willig and John Drury begin with a discourse on what is radical and limiting about a social constructionist perspective in critical psychology. They argue its main research tool, discourse analysis, still positions the researcher as an expert analyst who is superior to or stands outside the participants (the researched). This form of relational violence is inevitable as it is built into the class structure of all academic research activity and even characterizes action research in workplace settings. Here the authors present a unique collaborative research practice called *partisan participant observation*.

Partisan participant observation deconstructs the relational violence of an outside expert position in psychology research by encouraging researchers to consciously and actively position themselves within the social context under study. It involves taking sides and adopting the perspective and objectives of those one wishes to study. This is illustrated by the study of crowd events in social psychology. The authors present a fascinating hands-on account of partisan participant observation in relation to a crowd occupying the base of a chestnut tree during the building of the M11 link road in Wanstead, London, in 1993.

In this chapter, we introduce partisan participant observation as a way of addressing relational violence in social psychological research. We argue that while social constructionist approaches offer researchers a radical reappraisal of the nature of knowledge and understanding, they have not enabled them to challenge their own role as experts in the production of knowledge. As a result, we would argue, attempts to minimize relational violence have encountered obstacles. This chapter offers a structural conceptualization of relational violence that recognizes the researcher's positioning within the relations of power which characterize class society. Rather than attempting to escape from these, partisan participant observation allows the researcher to consciously and actively take sides within a social context and to adopt the perspective and objectives of those he or she wishes to study. In this way, relational violence as a structural phenomenon can be challenged through participation. The chapter provides an illustration of partisan participant observation research and concludes by pointing to future applications of the approach.

THE RADICAL IN SOCIAL CONSTRUCTIONISM . . .

Social constructionism draws our attention to possibilities. It reminds us that there is always more than one version of events, and that experiences can be read in different ways. Objects, subjects, phenomena, and experiences are made what they are by those who speak about and/or interact with them. They are social constructions rather than independent entities; they are created, rather than simply encountered, by social actors. This means that change is possible. If we do not like the version of reality that we have constructed, we can use our creative resources in order to transform it. Social constructionism opens up possibilities for change because it emphasizes our active participation in the construction of our world(s). Social constructionists make us think about the future as a creative project.

Social constructionist researchers have used forms of discourse analysis and deconstruction in order to challenge psychological concepts that serve ideological functions. For example, categories such as "intelligence," "personality," and "mental illness" have been reconceptualized as socioculturally and historically specific phenomena that are constructed through a range of discourses and practices and which perpetuate as well as legitimate existing social and economic divisions within society (see, for example, Henriques et al., 1984/1998; Parker et al., 1995; Rose, 1989/1999). In addition, social constructionist psychologists have reconceptualized "thinking" as a process that is inherently discursive and rhetorical (e.g., Billig et al., 1988; Edwards and Potter, 1992; Harre and Gillett, 1994) in that it requires a continuous engagement with and an orientation to (potential) counterclaims and challenges.

These constitute the context within which "thinking" takes place. As a result, social constructionist psychologists do not expect human cognition to be characterized by stability and consistency; instead, variability and contradiction are expected in relation to our attitudes and beliefs and even in relation to our sense of self and identity. Again, the flexibility and openness associated with social constructionist thought allows us to think about possibilities for change. People are conceptualized as actively engaging with their social environment and as capable of transformation as a result of this engagement. This is very different from an essentialist view, which sees the individual as being characterized by (and trapped within) stable and deep-rooted personality traits, gendered subjectivities, intelligence levels, susceptibilities to mental health/illness, and so on.

. . . AND SOME OF ITS LIMITATIONS

Although the turn to language and social constructionism enabled critical psychologists to formulate a radical critique of essentialism, it did not come without its own baggage. One of the most controversial aspects of social constructionist thought has been its fluidity. Social constructionism does not have a "bottom line" and it does not offer any certainties (e.g., Edwards, Ashmore, and Potter, 1995). If social constructionism is right and things do not have to be the way they are, and if contemporary versions of reality are constructed by discourses and practices which could conceivably be abandoned and replaced by their users, then "reality" as such does not exist independently of what we make of it. Furthermore, our own judgments about which of the various versions of "reality" is to be preferred are themselves the product of moral-political discourses which, in turn, are nothing more than historically and culturally specific social constructions. This implies that there is nothing that structurally preexists social constructions and gives them their texture and direction. Everything that is said, felt, and done by us is the product of our choice of which discourses and practices to engage with at a particular point in time.

Social constructionist researchers in psychology disagree about the extent to which individuals are free to choose which discursive constructions to deploy in their engagement with the social world (see Parker, 1998). However, the most widely used version of discourse analysis in psychology emphasizes the functionality of language. Such analysis is concerned with language use as a form of social action. As such, it constructs the speaker as rationally maximizing her or his personal interest—strategically deploying discourse in order to avoid blame, disclaim unwanted attributions, and generally manage the social world in self-serving ways. The subject of discursive psychology is, therefore, a close relation of *homo economicus,* familiar to liberal economic theory.

In addition, discourse analysis positions its practitioners as experts. This is because discourse analysis, when used as a research methodology within the context of academic research, presupposes a division of labor between the "participant" and the "analyst." The former produces the data while the latter unravels the participant's discursive constructions and positionings, and points to their functions and their contradictions. The result is a position of superiority for the researcher, whose analysis of participants' talk can, and often does, serve to mock speakers' self-serving versions of reality. Although this may be a legitimate weapon when we are researching those whose power we wish to undermine (e.g., politicians, various experts), it is certainly not an approach that is conducive to collaborative research with those whose experiences we wish to understand, appreciate, and also possibly enhance.

We would argue that relational violence is inevitable as long as the academic practitioner occupies the position of the expert.[1] Since academia positions *all* academics as experts, there is no way in which even the most critical of discourse analysts can sidestep relational violence within the academic framework.

RELATIONAL VIOLENCE AS A STRUCTURAL PHENOMENON

Thus, despite its radical approach to the production of knowledge, social constructionist research retains a traditional academic conceptualization of the relationship between researcher (as expert) and researched (as objects/subjects of the research). Other researchers in psychology have attempted to break out of the academic setting by using their expertise in the service of those who may benefit from it (e.g., in action research). However, they have tended to approach their subject matter from an individualistic perspective, according to which society comprises relations between individuals. As a result, attempts at challenging relational violence take the form of empowerment of individuals (to become more assertive, to gain voice, to learn new skills) through various forms of discursive and practical facilitation (e.g., Willig, 1999). However, an individualistic perspective, when applied, for example, to workplace action research, is unable to explain how the actors involved come to find themselves within given relationships of subordination and power.

An individualistic action research perspective is therefore ideological when it suggests individual solutions rather than recognizing power difference that derives from roles ("shop-floor worker," "manager," "employer," and so on) which are determined by a class society. What individualism fails to acknowledge, in other words, is that particular individuals are not *just* individuals but are also exemplars of broader *categories* of people—working class, managers, ruling class—who enter into such power relationships by their *category* nature. By extension, the individualistic approach also fails to engage with the role of the researcher and his or her positioning within such power relations. It says nothing, for example, about *why* the action researcher is being employed by the managers instead of being able to define a research agenda with the shop-floor workers.

Workplace action research in this kind of example is clearly a case of relational violence since workers and employers do not have an equal say in the nature of the research. But the example also points us to the necessity of a partial reconceptualization of relational violence which might, in turn, help us to be more reflective and critical in our own research. Just as class society defines the distinction, and hence power difference, between employer and worker, so the very nature of the expert role assumed by the action researcher needs to be understood in class terms. The distinction between expert and nonexpert expresses a division of labor through which human activity becomes part of the self-expansion of capital. The separation of most of humanity from its means of producing and consequently from its own product is only the (historically) most basic of a whole series of separations through which capital develops and humanity becomes impoverished.

Specialized expertise arises to de-skill and hence disempower workers through separating thinking from acting. The result is that de-skilled work loses its value, while the smaller group of experts—inheritors of the accumulated wisdom of generations of past workers—are able to command a relatively higher price or other privileges for their work. (This partly compensates them for their impoverished experience of life—"intellectual" rather than "practical.") Particular classes therefore play the roles of experts, and are able to employ such experts, while other people—that is, working-class people—are those typically pronounced upon by these same experts. Within such relationships, therefore, the power-difference that defines relational violence assumes a pattern—a structure. In short, patterns of relational violence are not just a function of the moral failings or lack of awareness on the part of individuals, but express class-based power difference.

PARTISAN PARTICIPANT OBSERVATION AS AN ATTEMPT TO MINIMIZE STRUCTURAL RELATIONAL VIOLENCE

One way that research might draw upon a structural reconceptualization of relational violence is to carry out partisan participant observation (PPO). PPO involves taking sides and adopting the perspective and objectives of those one wishes to study. One of us (John Drury) carried out a study into the self-definition of participants in a crowd event using PPO. This study thus constitutes an example of a form of research that at least attempts to minimize relational violence conceptualized in class (struggle) terms.

The background to this study is the role of historically dominant traditions within social psychology in abstracting crowd events from their social contexts (Reicher, 1987). Methodologically, this has been achieved through a reliance on partial secondary evidence (often recorded by observers hostile to the crowd) and, more recently, through the use of the laboratory experimental method. Both approaches separate the researcher from the researched, and have served to reify particular crowd behaviors as generic, thus precluding enquiry into participants' constructions of meaning within particular crowd events (see Drury and Stott, 2001).

The crowd event in question was an occupation against the building of the M11 link road in Wanstead, London, in 1993. Road building has been one way that capital expansion and profits are maintained (and hence ruling-class interests served). As a result, participation against the road meant support for the class (proletariat, broadly conceived) against whose interests the road was being built. PPO here therefore meant being on the side of those resisting the loss of houses and community resources such as green spaces. Indeed, one of the criteria for choosing the anti-road campaign for the research project was that it was one for which the researcher already had sympathies. As a "political subject," he would not have chosen to research a movement in which he would not have taken part anyway.

The event comprised a struggle involving the police attempting to remove crowd participants occupying the base of a chestnut tree scheduled to be demolished to make way for the road. The researcher had already been participating in campaign actions and collecting material for over a month previously. He participated in resisting the tree's removal by sitting down with the rest of the crowd and being forcibly ejected by police. He then remained with the crowd, which attempted to block the road contractors' vehicles and breach police lines for most of the rest of the event, which lasted around twelve hours.

Several hours of soundtrack recordings were made during the event and observations were recorded by hand or into a tape machine. It was also possible to interview participants immediately before the police arrival, during lulls in the actual conflict, and again in the days and weeks afterward. It was precisely because Drury was known personally to the antiroads participants as "one of that campaign" that people were willing to cooperate with him in these ways. It was significant that so many participants were willing to donate their time: fifty-six people were interviewed in relation to the event in question, several of them more than once. He was also given access to fifty-seven witness statements, as well as video recordings taken by participants, diary material, and campaign documents.

The researcher could not have expected people who were making such a commitment to the antiroad campaign to cooperate with him in these ways unless he was on their side. Why should they help the researcher unless he was helping them? If he were simply in it for his career, he would have been seen (correctly) as a parasite. So he helped the campaign not just by being one of the numbers in the collective actions, but also in more mundane ways such as folding leaflets and barricading buildings. Moreover, such involvement meant being in precisely the places where he could meet more campaign participants who could then help in the research.

Based on this research carried out within the PPO framework, according to which we take seriously participants' accounts as meaningful constructions of their social relations, we proposed a psychological model of identity-change through collective action. We argued that such change may come about when crowd participants act upon one understanding of self-and-world (e.g., "individual citizens engaging in legitimate peaceful protest") and yet are treated by a powerful "outgroup"—such as the police—in a way that contradicts this understanding (e.g., "dangerous mob") (Drury and Reicher, 2000). For more than a century, psychology has pathologized collective resistance by characterizing crowd events as atavistic and normless outbursts (e.g., Diener, 1980; Le Bon, 1895; Zimbardo, 1970). This has had the practical consequence of justifying repression of the crowd by the authorities (Reicher and Potter, 1985). Through the PPO framework, we were able to contribute to a broader project of countering such ideological characterizations of the crowd (Reicher, 1987, 1996, 2001; Stott and Reicher, 1998).

From the point of view of mainstream social psychology, participant observation is not a favored research method because the subjectivity of the researcher is thought to "contaminate" the research object. Against this we would argue that it is *because* we have subjectivity that we can develop understanding. However, from our own perspective, there were nevertheless a number of problems with the research.

First, to the extent that the researcher had to be able to get on with as many people as possible within the campaign in order to interview them, there was a certain amount of holding back on his own critical perspective. That is, he had usually to be nonjudgmental within the "in-group" of campaign participants, when he might otherwise (as a nonresearcher) have been more overtly critical. In taking sides against the road, the researcher obviously shared the "superordinate" identity and discourse of the protest community; but *within* this community there were also arguments and differences of emphasis about the essence of that shared identity. Two examples within the No M11 campaign that he might otherwise have openly criticized were tendencies to mysticism and to (ideological) nonviolence based on an individualistic principle.

A second limit is that of the narrowing of perspective that came about once the "data-gathering" phase was over and the write-up had to begin in earnest. PPO allowed a rich and fulfilling linking of theory and practice—taking sides in struggle, as Drury did, itself contributed to answering the research questions and simultaneously (he hoped) furthered the struggle. Yet the actual writing of a research paper (or in this case a doctoral thesis) necessarily means that many of the concerns operating for him at the time had to be bracketed off. He was no longer able to devote as much attention to the struggle against the expansion of capital through its ecologically destructive transport practices; instead he focused exclusively on narrower questions of psychological theory.

Third and finally, linking these two points, is the parasitism of academia upon one's subjectivity. At any one time, there may be a conflict between the need to "get stuck in" and the need to gather material for the research. The research project engenders a certain way of thinking and acting that is not always and necessarily that of the "active participant." Academia, as a realm of endless "words and ideas," draws heavily upon the researcher's mental and physical energy, using him or her up in order to produce material that is typically the purview of a small (inactive) minority.

CONCLUSION

The argument of this chapter is that, in order to minimize relational violence in psychological research, any method will have to acknowledge that we as researchers are positioned as subjects in relations of power and resistance. Therefore the issue is not whether PPO is superior to social constructionist discourse analysis, but how and when either is the appropriate research framework for a particular research problem.

We acknowledge that PPO cannot be applied to all topics. However, we will finish by suggesting an example of a possible research project that makes use of both PPO and discourse analysis. An obvious starting point for developing a critical research project—one that seeks to problematize given power relations—is one's own social location. Indeed, in the case of academics such as ourselves, the ongoing economic rationalization of the academic realm offers much to criticize and, hence, to research.

First, such a research project could be partisan and participatory in that it would be part of the resistance to the rationalization of the universities among both students and all levels of workers (academics, support staff, technicians). One strand of the research could comprise a form of support for students involved in occupations against tuition fees. For example, where university administrators seek to delegitimize and criminalize an occupation, researchers might document and analyzc psychologically positive aspects of the event, such as the subjective empowerment developed among participants.

Second, such research might also be social constructionist in that it would use discourse analysis to problematize the dominant instrumentalist discourses that are currently shaping the academic experience of both students and lecturers (see Fairclough, 1993). The economic rationalization of the university engenders consumerist subjectivities amongst students, who are encouraged to look at courses in terms of whether or not they offer value for money. University administrators likewise monetarize the functioning of the university through arguments within which financial considerations are characterized in terms of the "iron laws" of mathematics—in other words, a realm that excludes human intervention and which objectifies their own (rationalizing) role. Researchers might carry out discourse analysis on such materials as part of the "ideological battle" against the "inevitability" of rationalization.

We must add, finally, however, that there are obvious limits to academics' attempts to minimize relational violence, whether through PPO or discourse analysis. The separations and class divisions discussed above are nowhere more evident than in academia itself: academia is a realm of "knowledge," free from "practical" concerns, which positions its subjects as knowledge experts. There is no escape from the knowledge-expert role defined by academia unless academia itself is negated. Although we might be able to make moderate interventions within our roles, what ultimately is necessary is that we "act out of role." The key to challenging the whole system of roles and hence class-based patterns of relational violence lies in the possibility of the researcher assuming other subjectivities than that which defines her or him through her or his work/career.

Current disputes within academia over pay, conditions, and the future of education can illustrate the point. Striking academic researchers on picket lines find themselves in a relatively novel social location—relating to the university not just through a realm of ideas and arguments, but in terms of practical antagonism as they persuade their colleagues not to work. Hence, as the social value of the knowledge expert becomes financially devalued (even proletarianized to some degree), so other subjectivities become both possible and necessary, opening the way for academic researchers to see themselves as more like other groups sharing similar (antagonistic) relationships with those in power—including (lower paid) support staff and manual workers at the university. Hence a new form of collaboration becomes thinkable.

NOTE

1. Relational violence can be said to occur whenever a person's or a group's experiences are made sense of through categories or networks of meaning imposed upon them by others (see Larner, 1999; Paré, 1999). Relational violence is not necessarily experienced as harmful or damaging by those subjected to it and it is likely to be part of many, if not most, learning and socialization processes experienced by members of contemporary society.

REFERENCES

Billig, M., Condor, S., Edwards, D., Gane, M., Middleton, D., and Radley, A. (1988). *Ideological Dilemmas: A Social Psychology of Everyday Thinking*. London: Sage.
Diener, E. (1980). Deindividuation: The absence of self-awareness and self-regulation in group members. In P.B. Paulus (Ed.), *Psychology of Group Influence* (pp. 209-242). Hillsdale, NJ: Lawrence Erlbaum.
Drury, J. and Reicher, S. (2000). Collective action and psychological change: The emergence of new social identities. *British Journal of Social Psychology* 39: 579-604.
Drury, J. and Stott, C. (2001). "Bias" as a research strategy in participant observation: The case of intergroup conflict. *Field Methods* 14: 47-67.
Edwards, D., Ashmore, M., and Potter, J. (1995). Death and furniture: The rhetoric, politics and theology of bottom line arguments against relativism. *History of the Human Sciences* 8: 25-49.

Edwards, D. and Potter, J. (1992). *Discursive Psychology.* London: Sage.

Fairclough, N. (1993). Critical discourse analysis and the marketization of public discourse: The universities. *Discourse and Society* 4: 133-168.

Harre, R. and Gillett, G. (1994). *The Discursive Mind.* London: Sage.

Henriques, J., Hollway, W., Urwin, C., Venn, C., and Walkerdine, V. (1984/1998). *Changing the Subject: Psychology, Social Regulation and Subjectivity.* London: Routledge.

Larner, G. (1999). Derrida and the deconstruction of power as context and topic in therapy. In I. Parker (Ed), *Deconstructing Psychotherapy* (pp. 39-53). London: Sage.

Le Bon, G. (1895). *The Crowd: A Study of the Popular Mind.* London: Ernest Benn.

Paré, D. (1999). "Discursive Wisdom: Reflections on Ethics and Therapeutic Knowledge." Paper presented at Millenium World Conference on Critical Psychology, Sydney, New South Wales, Australia, May 2.

Parker, I. (Ed.) (1998). *Social Constructionism, Discourse and Realism.* London: Sage.

Parker, I., Georgaca, E., Harper, D., McLaughlin, T., and Stowell-Smith, M. (1995). *Deconstructing Psychopathology.* London: Sage.

Reicher, S.D. (1987). Crowd behavior as social action. In J.C. Turner, M.A. Hogg, P.J. Oakes, S.D. Reicher, and M.S. Wetherell (Eds.), *Rediscovering the Social Group: A Self-Categorization Theory* (pp. 171-202). Oxford: Blackwell.

Reicher, S.D. (1996). "The Battle of Westminster": Developing the social identity model of crowd behavior in order to explain the initiation and development of collective conflict. *European Journal of Social Psychology* 26: 115-134.

Reicher, S.D. (2001). The psychology of crowd dynamics. In M. Hogg and R.S. Tindale (Eds.), *The Blackwell Handbook of Social Psychology: Group Processes* (pp. 182-208). Oxford: Blackwell.

Reicher, S.D. and Potter, J. (1985). Psychological theory as intergroup perspective: A comparative analysis of "scientific" and "lay" accounts of crowd events. *Human Relations* 38: 167-189.

Rose, N. (1989/1999). *Governing the Soul: The Shaping of the Private Self.* London: Free Association Books.

Stott, C.J. and Reicher, S.D. (1998). Crowd action as inter-group process: Introducing the police perspective. *European Journal of Social Psychology* 28: 509-529.

Willig, C. (Ed.) (1999). *Applied Discourse Analysis: Social and Psychological Interventions.* Buckingham, UK: Open University Press.

Zimbardo, P.G. (1970). The Human Choice: Individuation, Reason and Order versus De-Individuation, Impulse and Chaos. In W.J. Arnold and D. Levine (Eds.), *Nebraska Symposium on Motivation 1969* (pp. 237-307). Lincoln: University of Nebraska.

SUGGESTED READINGS

Drury, J. and Stott, C. (2001). "Bias" as a research strategy in participant observation: The case of intergroup conflict. *Field Methods* 14: 47-67.

Willig, C. (Ed.) (1999). *Applied Discourse Analysis: Social and Psychological Interventions*. Buckingham, UK: Open University Press.

Chapter 18

Research and Solidarity: Partnerships for Knowing with Community Members

Isaac Prilleltensky
Geoffrey Nelson

This chapter presents collaborative research in psychology as a partnership or *knowing with* others that empowers its participants. It is informed by a politics of social justice where knowledge is used to enhance the wellness of persons who are marginalized, oppressed, and disadvantaged in society. In what the authors call solidarity research, values as moral guidelines for thought and action reenter the psychological domain and vocabulary. They identify a set of values to guide psychological research that promote the personal, collective, and relational wellness of persons in a community. These include: self-determination, health and personal growth, caring and compassion, social justice, support for enabling community structures, respect for diversity, and collaboration and democratic participation.

How these guidelines for solidarity research can be put into practice is discussed further. The first step is to decide who participates and how. It is here the radical social impact of solidarity research becomes evident as disadvantaged people actively plan and guide the project and carry it out as assistants with the support of trained community researchers. The authors make clear that well-defined procedures of decision-making and conflict resolution as well as for developing communication and networks of participation and connection are essential to the solidarity process. Two case examples of research partnerships are given, one involving Latin American refugee families and the other psychiatric consumers/survivors.

Together and separately we have worked with people who have been marginalized for different reasons, including psychiatric disabilities, refugee status, ethnic background, age, and gender. Although we have been trained in positivist paradigms that tend to objectify research participants, we have questioned and sought alternatives to them. We have witnessed research projects that have further victimized disempowered people. Our reaction has been anger and shame. Anger because in the name of knowledge we forget the person; shame because we are part of the professional world that has victimized people. However, following the anger and shame came creativity and opportunity. We have had chances to develop collaborative relationships with groups of people who wanted research to advance their own personal or collective welfare.

These research relationships gave us an opportunity to translate our community and critical psychology precepts into action (Nelson et al., 1998; Prilleltensky and Nelson, 1997). Our view of health and wellness is based on a fit between the needs of the person and the resources available in the environment. Material and psychological resources are largely determined by social structures and circumstances into which people are born. Access to these resources is contingent upon structures of justice or injustice, fairness or inequality, liberation or oppression. The connection between domination or emancipation and wellness has always been obvious to us, and has guided much of our work in research and practice in the clinical, educational, and community domains. We see our role as contributing to emancipatory research, at the personal, interpersonal, community, social, and political levels.

Our disillusionment with traditional psychological research came not only from its outcomes but also from the very process of inquiry. Often the processes would not involve participants in determining the aim of the research or would disregard their needs. In the worst cases, research processes caused damage to participants. This realization led us to be very mindful of not only the *why* and *what* of research but also of the *how.*

RESEARCH PARTNERSHIPS FOR SOLIDARITY

Although we value, for different reasons, both applied and basic research, we see our role as advancing knowledge that is useful to marginalized people (Nelson, Lord, and Ochocka, 2001). Research is a limited resource, and we choose to make use of it to promote the wellness of disadvantaged populations. People who are poor and disempowered rarely are the beneficiaries of the latest medical and social research because they lack power to pressure governments and funding bodies. Therefore, we wish to contribute our time and skills to populations that do not benefit as much from societal innovations. From a philosophical point of view, we see our collective fate bound with the fate of those who struggle. Research should benefit not just those who claim a powerful stake in the politics of research funding, but also those who remain silent through the process of research priority setting. To practice in ways that are both morally justifiable and practically effective we invoke the concept of partnerships.

We define research partnerships for solidarity as value-based relationships between researchers and disadvantaged people; relationships that should strive to advance the values of caring, compassion, community, health, self-determination, participation, power sharing, human diversity, and social justice for disadvantaged people, both in the processes and the outcomes of the partnership and in multiple contexts (Nelson, Prilleltensky and MacGillivary, 2001; Nelson et al., 2000). While the concept of partnership draws attention to values, relationships, and processes, partnerships can also lead to a bridging of ideas and perspectives.

We wish to be explicit about the social objective of our research. Our aim is to collaborate with oppressed people to facilitate the achievement of their social aims. Justice, a fair distribution of societal resources, the elimination of discriminatory policies, access to health care and social services, economic security, voice and choice, and respect for diversity are paramount values in the personal and collective wellness of marginalized groups. We strive to find ways to advance these principles in the process and outcome of our work. We seek an integration between our moral values and our research work.

The research approach that we are advocating rests on the traditions of participatory research and action research. Although participatory research and action research have historically had somewhat different emphases, more recently these traditions have been blended into a more unified approach (Nelson et al., 1998). Hill Collins (1993) describes participatory action research "as a way for researchers and oppressed people to join in solidarity to take collective action, both short and long term, for radical social change" (p. xiv). The values underlying participatory action research include self-determination, collaboration, democratic participation, and social justice (Nelson et al., 1998). The next question is why do we really need values in solidarity research work.

VALUES IN SOLIDARITY RESEARCH

Values are guidelines for thinking and acting in ways that are morally defensible. Even those who repudiate the talk of values in psychology, lest it contaminate its scientific purity, do so from a value-laden point of view: values belong in the moral domain, not in the scientific domain (Kendler, 1994). For us, obviously, there is no way to dichotomize values into morally valid or scientifically acceptable. As cognitive schemas that guide our behavior, values do permeate all we do; whereas as moral tenets, values should permeate all we do. Either way, values are inescapable (Fox and Prilleltensky, 1996).

We do not claim to have the definitive series of values, not at all. In fact, we have revised our conception of values to reflect new research, feedback, and thinking in this area (Prilleltensky, 1997). Values represent our point of departure, not an end point. We expect transparency with regard to people's beliefs about the social uses of their research. Unless we articulate with clarity our guiding principles, we inhibit communication and contribute to confusion.

The values we espouse for solidarity are meant to guide the very process of research partnerships, as well as their outcomes. In other words, the values we present guide the means and the ends of research partnerships for solidarity. In the past we have applied these values to teaching, research, consultation, and community practice (Nelson et al., 2000; Nelson, Lord, and Ochocka, 2001; Prilleltensky, Peirson, and Nelson, 1997). We draw on previous work and expand on the implications of our values for knowing with community members. Tables 18.1 and 18.2 present, respectively, our notions of preferred outcomes and preferred processes for research partnerships.

The values we propose can be classified into three groups: (a) *values for personal wellness* (e.g., self-determination, caring and compassion, health and personal growth) (b) *values for collective wellness* (e.g., social justice, support for community structures), and (c) *values for relational wellness* (e.g., respect for human diversity, collaboration and democratic participation), where wellness is defined as a positive state of affairs brought about by the satisfaction of personal, collective, and relational needs of a community (Prilleltensky, Nel-

TABLE 18.1. Preferred Outcomes of Research Partnerships for Solidarity

Values	Preferred Outcomes for Community Members
Personal Wellness	
Self-determination	Ability of community members to pursue their chosen goals in life *in consideration* of other people's needs
Health and personal growth	Opportunities to develop physical and emotional well-being through acquisition of skills and behavioral change *in consideration* of structural and economic factors impinging on the health of the population at large
Caring and compassion	Creation of community settings where people can give and receive caring and compassion, *in consideration* of the need to promote not only psychological support but also economic and material security
Collective Wellness	
Social justice	Fair allocation of bargaining powers, resources, and obligations in society *in consideration* of people's differential power, needs, and abilities
Support for community	Presence of vital structures that meet the needs of entire communities *in consideration* of the risks of curtailing individual freedoms and fostering conformity and uniformity
Relational Wellness	
Respect for diversity	Respect and appreciation for diverse social identities and unique oppressions *in consideration* of need for solidarity and risk of social fragmentation
Collaboration and democratic participation	Peaceful, respectful, and equitable processes of dialogue whereby citizens have meaningful input into decisions affecting their lives, *in consideration* of need to act and not just avoid conflicts

TABLE 18.2. Preferred Processes for Research Partnerships for Solidarity

Values	Preferred Processes for Partnerships with Community Members
Personal Wellness	
Self-determination	Facilitate opportunities for community members to have voice and choice in selection of research topic and administration of research project *in consideration* of the fact that they usually come to the partnership with less power
Health and personal growth	Create opportunities for community members to experience personal health and growth *in consideration* of the fact that they have different needs for health and growth
Caring and compassion	Establish an atmosphere of acceptance where people feel welcomed and appreciated *in consideration* of the fact that interpersonal conflict is likely to occur among different members of the partnerships
Collective Wellness	
Social justice	Promote equal access to resources brought about by the research partnership, *in consideration* of the fact that it is usually researchers who get paid to do the research and who benefit from publications and personal promotion
Support for community	Foster processes that benefit not only the individual community partners but also the community at large by involving community organizations, *in consideration* of the fact that organizations can inhibit emancipation of individuals and collectives
Relational Wellness	
Respect for diversity	Create processes that recognize the ability and right of individuals to define their identity, *in consideration* of the risk that accentuating differences can diminish solidarity
Collaboration and democratic participation	Create tangible opportunities for community partners to express their needs and desires, *in consideration* of their relative lack of power vis à vis professional researchers

son, and Peirson, 2001). These categories of values reflect the need to balance individual and social goals, as well as the need for dialogue in resolving conflicts of interests. There is a dialectic between personal and collective values; one kind cannot exist without the other. But while this dialectic has been amply recognized (e.g., Bauman, 1993; Sandel, 1996), what is often missed in the literature is the need for relational values that mediate between the good of the individual and the good of the collective, a need that is often invoked in feminist (Hill Collins, 1993) and native writings (Gunn Allen, 1993), but that is rarely discussed in mainstream social philosophy. Neither personal nor collective values can exist without mechanisms for connecting between them (Habermas, 1990; Putnam, 1996).

There cannot be a *single* value that can promote personal, collective, and relational wellness. Rather, we need a *set* of values that is internally consistent, that avoids dogmatism and relativism, and that promotes congruence between means and ends. Whereas some values may advocate personal more than collective wellness, such as the principle of self-determination, others may balance it by fostering caring and compassion for others. This reasoning calls for a search for values that can balance the promotion of personal wellness with the affirmation of collective and relational wellness at the same time. Guided by such a call, we can identify a set of values that work in concert to meet the criteria established above: self-determination, health and personal growth, caring and compassion, social justice, support for enabling community structures, respect for diversity, and collaboration and democratic participation.

Table 18.1 states the preferred outcomes of each value and points to their interdependence. To emphasize the interdependence and synergy of the various values, each one of them asserts an objective *in consideration* of other values and types of wellness. In concert, these values promote personal, collective, and relational wellness. For example, the objective of *respect for diversity* is to promote respect and appreciation for diverse social identities and unique oppressions *in consideration* of the need for solidarity and risk of social fragmentation. Respect and appreciation for diverse identities promotes personal and collective wellness of individuals and a group, while solidarity with other groups fosters relational wellness and sensitivity to the collective wellness of other communities.

GUIDELINES FOR SOLIDARITY RESEARCH

Although solidarity research sounds conceptually and ideologically appealing to researchers and community members with an orientation towards social change, translating the ideals of this approach into action often is quite challenging. Through our experiences working on different projects with different groups of stakeholders, we have learned that it is useful to have practical guidelines to implement solidarity research. Solidarity research is not a completely open-ended process without boundaries. Like any research project, solidarity research has objectives and questions, methods and timeliness for data collection and analysis, and interpretation, report writing, and dissemination of findings. What distinguishes solidarity research from more traditional social science research is *how* these different steps and tasks are carried out. In this section, we outline some practical guidelines for conducting solidarity research.

Representation, Roles, and Responsibilities

We have argued elsewhere (Nelson et al., 2000) that the first step in a collaborative research project is to decide who should be "at the table." Based on the values of self-determination, collaboration, and democratic participation outlined in previous sections, we believe that the disadvantaged group that is the focus of the research should be strongly represented in the research process (Nelson, Prilleltensky, and MacGillivary, 2001). Depending on the focus of the research project, the research may be comprised solely of researchers and members of the disadvantaged group (e.g., a study of self-help organizations), or there may be wider stakeholder representation, including service providers, family members, and/or policy-makers and planners (e.g., a study of mental health reform). To help actualize substantial and meaningful participation of disadvantaged people in the research process, we suggest having a guideline of a minimum of 51 percent participation from the disadvantaged group.

It is also desirable to clarify the roles and responsibilities of those involved in the research (Butterfoss, Goodman, and Wandersman, 1993; Curtis and Hodge, 1994). In our projects, disadvantaged people typically participate in one of two ways: steering and guiding the project or actually carrying out the research. We have found it useful to create different structures for these different types of participation (Nelson et al., 1998). A research steering committee can be formed to oversee the development and implementation of the project, with representatives functioning somewhat like board members, making broad policy decisions. A research team, on the other hand, is responsible for carrying out the research, including collecting and analyzing the data.

In our research projects, steering committee representatives typically advocate for hiring members of the disadvantaged community to serve as research assistants. For those people who are hired as research assistants, the training, supervision, and experience that they obtain helps to facilitate their health and personal growth. Also, the steering committee can either act on its own behalf or it can link with other groups to use the research findings for advocacy and social change. These are ways in which solidarity research can be used to enact the value of social justice (Nelson et al., 1998).

With regard to the issue of representation, the roles and responsibilities of the community researchers are to help organize and provide a framework for the research, to solicit and encourage participation of the disadvantaged group in the research, and facilitate the clarification of roles and responsibilities of different participants. There are some tensions in ensuring representation. It is often difficult to decide who to include and who not to include. To keep the numbers manageable, sometimes not all individuals or organizations can be reasonably included. We have found it useful to provide other ways for people who do not participate on the project steering committee to have input on the project (e.g., inviting people to a community forum or consultation).

One of the first tasks of both the steering committee and research team is to brainstorm the vision, values, and working principles for the research project. Developing shared values and principles among partners is critical for successful solidarity partnerships (see Nelson, Prilleltensky, and MacGillivary, 2001). One essential part of the vision, values, and principles of a solidarity research project is that of decision making and conflict resolution, which is what we discuss next.

Decision-Making Power and Conflict Resolution

To implement the values of self-determination, collaboration, and democratic participation, it is also important to develop guidelines regarding decision-making power and conflict resolution. We believe that it is important to have not only the key parties "at the table" but also to have all aspects of the research "on the table" for discussion. Early in the process, the research steering committee must come up with guidelines for decision making (Nelson, Prilleltensky, and MacGillivary, 2001).

We have found it useful to come up with written guidelines or procedures for conflict resolution. Conflict is an inevitable part of any interpersonal process and having guidelines in place as to how to handle such conflict is useful for preventing conflict escalation (Butterfoss, Goodman, and Wandersman, 1993; Nelson, Prilleltensky, and MacGillivary, 2001). Addressing whatever conflict arises quickly and with clear and direct communication is helpful in minimizing any potential damage that could ensue. The role of the community researcher with respect to issues of decision making and conflict is to share power and to help facilitate conflict resolution. Power and conflict are essentially relational in nature. Thus, it is important to consider guidelines for the types of relationships that are desired in solidarity research.

Communication and Supportive Relationships

Whenever we develop working principles for solidarity research with members of disadvantaged groups, the themes of communication and supportive relationships are always of paramount importance. Clear communication entails regular and direct communication among all participants, speaking for oneself, and using language that is accessible and free of jargon (Nelson, Prilleltensky, and MacGillivary, 2001). We have found that the structures of a research steering committee and a research team, which meet regularly to share information, are important vehicles for communication. However, it is also necessary to have methods of communication that go beyond the core research committees so that information can be shared more broadly. Steering committee members and research assistants play an important liaison role with their organizations, so that there can be more widespread sharing of information. Having periodic summary bulletins, news reports, and feedback sessions on the project are other valuable methods of communication. The more information that is shared in solidarity research, the more there is mutual ownership over the project.

We have found it useful in initial meetings to have people share some of their interests and hobbies, rather than talking about what their title is or what organization they represent. Such activities are useful in "breaking the ice" and helping people to make connections with one another. Part of the respect that disadvantaged people want is acknowledgment of the validity of their experiences and knowledge. Oftentimes professionals utilize research or professional knowledge and dismiss the experience of the people they serve. In solidarity research, there is an emphasis on mutual learning, learning as an ongoing process, and valuing the experiential knowledge of disadvantaged people (Nelson et al., 1998). To this end, qualitative methods that amplify the voices of disadvantaged people are often used in this type of research (Lord and Hutchison, 1993; Nelson, Prilleltensky, and MacGillivary, 2001).

We see the role of the researcher as creating a welcoming atmosphere for participation and facilitating communication and supportive relationships among team members. When people from disadvantaged groups feel comfortable and free to express their opinions and participate, the spirit of collaboration is realized.

CASE EXAMPLES

Partnership with Refugee Families

Beginning in 1991, while working at Wilfrid Laurier University, I (Isaac) started collaborating with a group of Latin American refugee families in Kitchener-Waterloo, Ontario, Canada. The partnership continued until 1997. The objective was to improve the educational and personal opportunities of children of refugees. The families lived in a cooperative housing with about eighty units, and Latin American families occupied about a quarter of them. Parents had been concerned about schools' responsiveness to their children's needs and came together to form the Latin American Educational Group.

In order to determine children's needs, we conducted a needs and resources assessment. With collaboration from community leaders we constructed an interview guide inquiring about risk and protective factors facing children and families in this refugee community. I trained community members in interviewing and focus group facilitation. Several parents helped with the research, including analysis and interpretation. The findings were conceptualized at various levels of analysis. Risk, protective factors, and recommendations were all discussed at the levels of child, family, school, and community (Prilleltensky, 1993). We presented together at several conferences and community forums.

Two of the central problems that were identified were the need to prevent smoking and the need to promote the Spanish language skills of children. Throughout the six years of this collaboration I worked closely with a steering committee to plan community-based research and evaluation of the various programs they implemented (Prilleltensky, Nelson, and Sanchez, 2000). The work with the Latin American community led to several prevention and promotion programs. Multiple needs called for multiple interventions, at various levels, and with various players. At the level of the child, there was a need to maintain the cultural heritage. This prompted the creation of a Spanish school run by parent volunteers. At the family level, there was a need for parenting courses, which were coordinated by local facilitators. At the school level, advocacy was needed to help educators understand the unique circumstances of refugee children from Latin America. This led to presentations and meetings with school board officials. At the level of the community, smoking prevention was seen as a priority. With government funding, a local initiative was launched to prevent smoking in children and youth. This program was not limited to skills but incorporated a community action component. Children made presentations at city hall concerning the ill effects of smoking and displayed antismoking art in a shopping center. All these activities were carried out in the spirit of action research and formative evaluations were often undertaken to see if the values of the group were being enacted in practice (Prilleltensky, Nelson, and Sanchez, 2000).

Partnerships with Psychiatric Consumer/Survivors

I (Geoff) have been working with psychiatric consumer/survivors for more than fifteen years. This work has included advocacy with consumer/survivors for housing and human rights, participatory action research with consumer/survivor self-help/mutual aid organizations, and forming a partnership with a community mental health agency and two consumer/survivor organizations to address the economic needs of consumer/survivors through supported employment and a loan fund.

In 1995, the Social Sciences and Humanities Research Council of Canada put out a call for research proposals which would involve partnerships between researchers and people with disabilities to examine issues of social and economic integration of people with disabilities. My colleagues, John Lord and Joanna Ochocka, and I met and talked about submitting a proposal for this competition. As we thought about what the focus of the study might be, we reflected on our experiences of community mental health services and supports in our home community of Waterloo Region. Since 1991, we had witnessed the emergence of a strong consumer/survivor self-help/mutual aid organization (Waterloo Region Self Help) and significant changes in two community mental health organizations (the Canadian Mental Health Association/Waterloo Region Branch and Waterloo Regional Homes for Mental Health). We were curious about the breadth and depth of the changes that we had seen and wondered if we were witnessing a shift from the traditional mental health paradigm to some alternative paradigm.

We knew each of these organizations and people within them quite well, and we approached the executive directors of the three organizations for a meeting to see if they would be interested in participating in a research study with us that would examine changes within their organizations. There was interest and we continued to meet with them over the summer to work on the proposal, which eventually got submitted and a few months later was successfully reviewed and funded.

At our first steering committee meeting, a representative from Waterloo Region Self Help asked us "well-paid professionals" if there was any money in the budget to hire consumer/survivors to work on this project. We did make such a plan and followed through by hiring, training, and supervising one consumer/survivor research assistant from each of the three settings. As we started the first phase of data collection, other representatives from Waterloo Region Self Help told us that the interview guide that we developed for the three agencies would not work so well for their setting. We worked with them to develop a more suitable guide.

We quickly realized that we were learning a great deal just from the process of doing this type of participatory action research. During our first training session for consumer/survivor research assistants, one of the people we hired asked to start the meeting with his view of empowerment. I remember this situation vividly—how eloquently this person spoke about the power loss and "spoiled identity" that he and other consumer/survivors experience and how empowerment is about having a voice and having choices. This person and the other research assistants went on to enrich this project in many ways and to benefit from it as well.

I learned how important it is to have consumer/survivors actively participate in all facets of a research project and to share power with them. As my colleagues and I gave up some of the power that typically rests with researchers, several consumer/survivors stepped up and exerted leadership and took responsibility for some of the work of the project.

At the beginning of the project, I had no idea that consumer/survivors would end up analyzing some of the data, writing up findings, and presenting the research at professional conferences with the researchers. For those who are interested in learning more of the particulars of this research project, I refer you to *Shifting the Paradigm in Community Mental Health* (Nelson, Lord, and Ochocka, 2001).

CONCLUSION

We have presented some broad guidelines for solidarity research based on our experiences and those of others reported in the literature. These guidelines can be helpful strategies for putting the values that we described into practice in community research projects. However, at the same time, it is important to realize that these guidelines are not offered as a step-by-step recipe. Improvisation, creativity, and being willing and open to respond to challenges to one's integrity are essential. Above all else, we are calling for a personal paradigm shift for researchers, a shift toward inclusion, power sharing, and supportive relationships with disadvantaged people in the research process.

As the case examples show, this type of research can be adopted by all researchers. There is nothing mystifying about it. In fact, we would like to encourage psychologists and other social scientists to venture into the community and to dialogue with people about their needs and research interests. In both case studies, community members enriched the research and contributed to knowledge.

REFERENCES

Bauman, Z. (1993). *Postmodern ethics*. Cambridge, MA: Blackwell.

Butterfoss, F. D., Goodman, R. M., and Wandersman, A. (1993). Community coalitions for prevention and health promotion. *Health Education Research* 8: 315-330.

Curtis L. C. and Hodge, M. (1994). Old standards, new dilemmas: Ethics and boundaries in community support services. *Psychosocial Rehabilitation Journal* 18(2): 13-33.

Fox, D. and Prilleltensky, I. (1996). The inescapable nature of politics in psychology. *New Ideas in Psychology 14*(1): 21-26.

Gunn Allen, P. (1993). Who is your mother? Red roots of White Feminism. In C. Lemert (Ed.), *Social theory: The multicultural and classic readings* (pp. 649-665). San Francisco: Westview.

Habermas, J. (1990). *Moral consciousness and communicative action*. Cambridge, MA: MIT Press.

Hill Collins, P. (1993). Black feminist thought in the matrix of domination. In C. Lemert (Ed.), *Social theory: The multicultural and classic readings* (pp. 615-626). San Francisco: Westview.

Kendler, H. H. (1994). Can psychology reveal the ultimate values of humankind? *American Psychologist* 49: 970-971.

Lord, J. and Hutchison, P. (1993). The process of empowerment: Implications for theory and practice. *Canadian Journal of Community Mental Health 12*(1): 5-22.

Nelson, G., Amio, J., Prilleltensky, I., and Nickels, P. (2000). Partnerships for implementing school and community prevention programs. *Journal of Educational and Psychological Consultation* 11: 121-145.

Nelson, G., Lord, J., and Ochocka, J. (2001). *Shifting the paradigm in community mental health: Towards empowerment and community*. Toronto, Canada: University of Toronto Press.

Nelson, G., Ochocka, J., Griffin, K., and Lord, J. (1998). "Nothing about me without me:" Participatory action research with self-help/mutual aid groups for psychiatric consumer/survivors. *American Journal of Community Psychology* 26: 881-912.

Nelson, G., Prilleltensky, I., and McGillivary, H. (2001). Value-based partnerships: Toward solidarity with oppressed groups. *American Journal of Community Psychology* 29: 649-678.

Prilleltensky, I. (1993). The immigration experience of Latin-American families: Research and action on perceived risk and protective factors. *Canadian Journal of Community Mental Health* 12(2): 101-116.

Prilleltensky, I. (1997). Values, assumptions, and practices: Assessing the moral implications of psychological discourse and action. *American Psychologist* 47: 517-535.

Prilleltensky, I. and Nelson, G. (1997). Community psychology: Reclaiming social justice. In D. Fox and I. Prilleltensky (Eds.), *Critical psychology: An introduction* (pp. 166-184). London: Sage.

Prilleltensky, I., Nelson, G., and Peirson, L. (Eds.) (2001). *Promoting family wellness and preventing child maltreatment.* Toronto, Canada: University of Toronto Press.

Prilleltensky, I., Nelson, G., and Sanchez, L. A. (2000). A value-based smoking prevention program with Latin American youth: Program evaluation. *Journal of Ethnic and Cultural Diversity in Social Work* 9(1-2): 97-117.

Prilleltensky, I., Peirson, L., and Nelson, G. (1997). The application of community psychology values and guiding concepts to school consultation. *Journal of Educational and Psychological Consultation* 8: 153-173.

Putnam, R. W. (1996). Creating reflective dialogue. In S. Toulmin and B. Gustavsen (Eds.), *Beyond theory: Changing organizations through participation* (pp. 41-52). Philadelphia, PA: John Benjamins.

Sandel, M. (1996). *Democracy's discontent.* Cambridge, MA: Harvard University Press.

SUGGESTED READINGS

Brydon-Miller, M. and Tolman, D. (Eds.) (1997). Transforming psychology: Interpretive and participatory research methods. *Journal of Social Issues* [Special issue] 53: 597-827.

MacGillivary, H. and Nelson, G. (1998). Partnership in mental health: What it is and how to do it. *Canadian Journal of Rehabilitation* 12: 71-83.

Park, P., Brydon-Miller, M., Hall, B., and Jackson, T. (Eds.) (1993). *Voices of change: Participatory research in the United States and Canada.* Westport, CT: Bergen and Garvey.

Reason, P. and Bradbury, H. (Eds.) (2001). *Handbook of action research: Participative inquiry and practice.* London: Sage.

Stringer, E. T. (1996). *Action research: A handbook for practitioners.* Thousand Oaks, CA: Sage.

Glossary

abjection: A term used with most resonance in the work of Julia Kristeva to indicate the experience of falling away or disappearing into a boundary state, a place of rupture or "corporeal abyss" out of which the subject is formed.

constructivism: A view of cognition, perception, and meaning that emphasizes the role of the individual observer in the construction of the thing perceived. Although related to social constructionism, constructivism places less emphasis on the social negotiation of meaning and attends instead to the individual's beliefs and predispositions in shaping experience.

deconstruction: A method of critique and reflective inquiry into traditions and institutions that opens up multiple meanings or alternative readings within texts, social practices, and conversations. Deconstruction leads to an unpacking and reevaluation of taken-for-granted meanings.

deconstructive questions: From narrative therapy; questions informed by a curiosity about the wider social meanings that undergird beliefs and behavior. Deconstructive questions uncover the latticework of cultural understandings that action is founded upon.

discursive: From the study of discourse and discourse analysis; when language, conversation, and therapy are regarded with a discursive focus, attention is paid to how talk operates to achieve certain results. A discursive view of therapy depicts the process as the negotiation of meaning through conversation, highlighting the exchange of individual utterances.

essential self: The modern idea that the self is an internal reality or essential entity and this subject is the causal agent behind thinking and behavior. Essentialism is typically associated with an individualist view of self, and can be contrasted with views that place greater emphasis on context, society, and culture.

externalization: A linguistic convention informed by ethical position, from narrative therapy. Externalizing conversations help to counter psychological traditions of pathologizing persons. They do this by speaking about the difficulties that clients face as separate from their identities.

instrumentalist discourse: Instrumentalist discourses are those in which categories, concepts, and criteria reflect concerns with "usefulness," and presume that every activity should serve as some tool or instrument and hence be judged as such. An instrumental orientation to others promotes a posture of "acting on" rather than "working with."

positivism: A philosophy of science, associated with modernism, which purports that valid knowledge is achieved through rational, objective, and value-free method. Positivist approaches emphasize facts and neutrality and can be contrasted with interpretivist approaches, which attend more to subjectivity, meaning, and perspective.

postmodernism: A contemporary movement throughout the humanities and social sciences characterized by a reaction against enlightenment era ideals of progress through the technical application of expert knowledge. In psychology and therapy, a postmodern orientation downplays formal categorization of such things as developmental stages or mental disorders, and emphasizes processes of mutual meaning-making and collaborative relationship.

rationalization: Rationalization refers to that tendency in economies, businesses, and publicly funded organizations to become more "efficient" through shedding "surplus" posts, cutting costs, and generally orienting more toward market considerations than social issues and needs.

realist epistemology: The notion that the world has a real existence independent of human knowing. A realist view can be contrasted with some forms of constructivism and constructionism that emphasize the way in which the world is constructed by individuals and collectives through perception and meaning-making.

reauthoring: From narrative therapy; the therapeutic process of reclaiming a story about one's identity that is aligned with one's values and commitments. Reauthoring conversations focus on and thicken descriptions of preferred developments in clients' lives.

reflexivity: A self-observing, mindful orientation. In a posture of reflexivity, we attend not only to that which is before us but also turn the mirror back on ourselves.

social constructionism: A philosophical position or worldview that attends to the ways meaning is constructed in a social and historical context. At the macrolevel, social constructionism looks at broad cultural discourse and how that discourse shapes both collective and individual meaning. At the microlevel, social constructionism emphasizes the dialogic feature of meaning-making: how the message communicated is always a function of speaker *and* listener.

speech-acting: This phrase highlights the active and constructive aspect of language. To speak is not merely to reflect the world or describe it, but to *do* something. Talk is action, and speaking is acting.

Name Index

Subject Index

Expert *(continued)*
  models, 161
  subjects as, 238
  position, 125, 229, 232
  stance, 23, 112
Expertise, 1, 2, 50, 55, 57, 60, 89, 112,
       151, 157, 161, 171, 187, 234
  client, 113-114, 176
  located in instructor, 145
  researcher, 232
  student, 126, 148
Externalization, 231, 260

Face, 77-79
Family story, 116
Family systems theory, 56
Family systems therapy, *see also*
      Therapy, family
Feedback
  questions, 93-94, 96
  from service consumers, 162
Feminist analysis, 184
Flexibility, *xxvi,* 19, 162, 223, 231

Gender
  bias, 57
  moral questions, 136-137
  solidarity research, 243
  in supervision, 183-185, 189-190,
    196
Generous listening, 32-33

Harassment, 121-122, 124, 127, 130
Harmonizing with clients, 94
Hierarchical practices, 148
Homo economicus, 232
Human nature, 10, 23, 46, 148,
    152-153, 201

Ideology, 2, 146
Imposability, 1

Individualism, *xxv,* 11, 18, 20, 233
Institutional humility, 3
Intersubjectivity, 62
Intervision, 183

Joint action, 214, 217

Kleinian theory, 62
Knowing
  bodily, 86, 88-89
  collaborative, 3
  four ways of, 87-89
  monologic, *xxvi*
  rational, 88-89
  relational, 88-89
  technical, 88-89
Knowing-that, 3, 121
Knowing-with, 3, 41, 97, 121, 133,
    157, 243
Knowledge
  adult, 124
  claims, 151, 181
  client, 150
  discoverers of, 124, 126
  experiential, 253
  expert, *xxvi,* 122, 125, 159, 162,
    66, 238, 260
  indigenous, 126
  invoking of, 145
  legitimation of, 145
  "of practice," 160
  practice-based, 157, 160
  production of, 230, 232
  professional, 60, 176, 181, 253
  psychological, 157
  relationship to, 150
  research-based, 160
  student, 126, 148
  student mediation, 126
  therapeutic, 113
  transmitting of, 145
  young people's, 124

SPECIAL 25%-OFF DISCOUNT!

Order a copy of this book with this form or online at:
http://www.haworthpress.com/store/product.asp?sku=4853

COLLABORATIVE PRACTICE IN PSYCHOLOGY AND THERAPY

_____in hardbound at $44.96 (regularly $59.95) (ISBN: 0-7890-1785-7)

_____in softbound at $26.21 (regularly $34.95) (ISBN: 0-7890-1786-5)

Or order online and use special offer code HEC25 in the shopping cart.

COST OF BOOKS_____

OUTSIDE US/CANADA/
MEXICO: ADD 20%_____

POSTAGE & HANDLING_____
*(US: $5.00 for first book & $2.00
for each additional book)*
*(Outside US: $6.00 for first book
& $2.00 for each additional book)*

SUBTOTAL_____

IN CANADA: ADD 7% GST_____

STATE TAX_____
*(NY, OH, MN, CA, IN, & SD residents,
add appropriate local sales tax)*

FINAL TOTAL_____
*(If paying in Canadian funds,
convert using the current
exchange rate, UNESCO
coupons welcome)*

☐ **BILL ME LATER:** ($5 service charge will be added)
(Bill-me option is good on US/Canada/Mexico orders only;
not good to jobbers, wholesalers, or subscription agencies.)

☐ Check here if billing address is different from
shipping address and attach purchase order and
billing address information.

Signature_____

☐ **PAYMENT ENCLOSED: $**_____

☐ **PLEASE CHARGE TO MY CREDIT CARD.**

☐ Visa ☐ MasterCard ☐ AmEx ☐ Discover
☐ Diner's Club ☐ Eurocard ☐ JCB

Account # _____

Exp. Date_____

Signature_____

Prices in US dollars and subject to change without notice.

NAME_____

INSTITUTION_____

ADDRESS_____

CITY_____

STATE/ZIP_____

COUNTRY_____ COUNTY (NY residents only)_____

TEL_____ FAX_____

E-MAIL_____

May we use your e-mail address for confirmations and other types of information? ☐ Yes ☐ No
We appreciate receiving your e-mail address and fax number. Haworth would like to e-mail or fax special
discount offers to you, as a preferred customer. **We will never share, rent, or exchange your e-mail address
or fax number.** We regard such actions as an invasion of your privacy.

Order From Your Local Bookstore or Directly From
The Haworth Press, Inc.
10 Alice Street, Binghamton, New York 13904-1580 • USA
TELEPHONE: 1-800-HAWORTH (1-800-429-6784) / Outside US/Canada: (607) 722-5857
FAX: 1-800-895-0582 / Outside US/Canada: (607) 771-0012
E-mailto: orders@haworthpress.com
PLEASE PHOTOCOPY THIS FORM FOR YOUR PERSONAL USE.
http://www.HaworthPress.com   BOF03